# Praise for

# HEALING WITH THE ARTS

"*Healing with the Arts* lays out a program of transformation through the union of creative and healing forces. This inner alchemy is a pure spiritual practice and this book is a map toward a healthy life you love."

**—Alex Grey and Allyson Grey**, artists,
cofounders of Chapel of Sacred Mirrors,
and coauthors of *Net of Being*

"*Healing with the Arts* is an exceptional guide to the power of art in deep intentional healing. Michael Samuels and Mary Rockwood Lane are leaders in the field. I recommend their book strongly."

**—Michael Lerner**, president of Commonweal

"This twelve-week program uses art to heal; it is based on two simple premises: art is the most powerful healing force we know; and everyone of us has both an inner artist and an inner healer. Read this book and discover for yourself the simple but profound truths it contains."

**—John Graham-Pole, MD, MRCP-UK**,
emeritus professor, University of Florida College of Medicine
cofounder of Arts in Medicine, Shands Hospital

"Every day I bear witness to the creativity that lies within each and every person. *Healing with the Arts* offers the possibility of transformation through one's own self-process."

**—Cynthia D. Perlis**, director of Art for Recovery
UCSF Helen Diller Family Comprehensive Cancer Center

"*Healing with the Arts* is a guidebook for everyone, not just artists, or patients in the healthcare setting."

**—Cathy DeWitt**, national consultant for the
Society for the Arts in Healthcare

"Through the elegance, depth, and insight of Mary and Michael's writings, the reader is guided through a process that can help them unlock their most inner truth, the one that can ultimately set us free, free to be ourselves and to be fulfilled once again.

**—Robert Browning**,
healthcare director for HeartMath

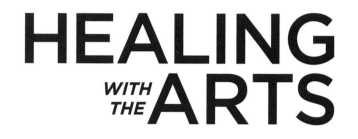

# HEALING
## WITH THE ARTS

# HEALING
## WITH THE ARTS

## A 12-Week Program to Heal Yourself and Your Community

**MICHAEL SAMUELS, MD,** and
**MARY ROCKWOOD LANE, PHD, RN**

**ATRIA** PAPERBACK
New York London Toronto Sydney New Delhi

BEYOND WORDS
Hillsboro, Oregon

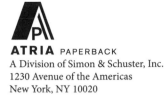

**ATRIA** PAPERBACK
A Division of Simon & Schuster, Inc.
1230 Avenue of the Americas
New York, NY 10020

**BEYOND** WORDS
20827 N.W. Cornell Road, Suite 500
Hillsboro, Oregon 97124-9808
503-531-8700 / 503-531-8773 fax
www.beyondword.com

Managing editor: Lindsay S. Brown
Editors: Henry Covey and Emily Han
Copyeditor: Claire Rudy Foster
Proofreader: Jade Chan
Interior Design: Devon Smith
Composition: William H. Brunson Typography Services

First Atria Paperback/Beyond Words trade paperback edition November 2013

For more information about special discounts for bulk purchases, please contact Simon & Schuster Special Sales at 1-866-506-1949 or business@simonandschuster.com.

The Simon & Schuster Speakers Bureau can bring authors to your live event. For more information or to book an event, contact the Simon & Schuster Speakers Bureau at 1-866-248-3049 or visit our website at www.simonspeakers.com.

Manufactured in the United States of America

10 9 8 7 6 5 4 3 2 1

*Library of Congress Cataloging-in-Publication Data:*

Samuels, Michael.
    Healing with the arts : a 12-week program to heal yourself and your community / Michael Samuels, MD, PhD, Mary Rockwood Lane, PhD, RN, FAAN.
       pages   cm
1. Art therapy.   I. Lane, Mary Rockwood.   II. Title.
RC489.A7S26   2013
616.89'1656—dc23
                                                                    2013019305

ISBN 978-1-58270-393-0
ISBN 978-1-4516-9683-7 (ebook)

*The corporate mission of Beyond Words Publishing, Inc.: Inspire to Integrity*

I dedicate this book to Danielle Ory for her love and support in my life.
*Michael*

I dedicate this to book to Jean Watson for our friendship and for the inspiration of her human caring theory, my foundation for art and healing.
*Mary*

Together, we both dedicate this book to the reader,
to the artist and healer you are.

May you open your heart and experience the beauty of art and healing.

# CONTENTS

# FOREWORD

This book brings art and healing to life in ways that are unique and purposeful for anyone and everyone. Michael Samuels, MD, and Mary Rockwood Lane, PhD, RN, use their world-class experiences and expertise to create and implement revolutionary medical arts programs in the United States. Using their own personal and professional experiences, they bring forth healing with the arts as a twelve-week program for you, the reader, and us and our community, wherever we may find ourselves.

The exercises in this book entice us into new space, meaning, and dimensions that touch on the holy, the sacred, as they guide the reader into deep inner territory. We rediscover light and dark parts of our being and become whole, holy, and healed.

How do they do this? They teach us to be our own best artist, expressing the artistry of shared humanity and uncovering our human spirit, the source of creativity. We reconsider the meaning of art—that is, art as anything that brings creativity, beauty, love, and light into our life. Anything that invites more light into the inner darkness associated with vast vicissitudes of all our human existence, of all our human frailties and detours from Source and spirit, using art to bring us home to the sacred heart, the very source of divine Love.

*Healing with the Arts* transcends the usual approach to healing and to art. It is a culmination of the authors' life works and personal practices. Michael and Mary search for the source of spirit, using their creative existence to come closer to the sacred. These practices transcend "sense" and mainstream mind-sets. The authors use self as instruments for the artist's way. We become sojourners on their path into deeper healing and awakening of the soul. They embrace the freedom and emancipation of the human spirit, uninhibited on the journey to oneness.

Through the authors' poetic, visual, and lyrical approach to life processes, you can heal yourself. You can transcend old patterns, find your inner essence, and journey forward to fulfill your life's work, purpose, and destiny.

Michael and Mary share their own healing journeys through art: Mary painted her way through depression, and Michael healed a patient's arthritic pain via illustration. I, too, have experienced the inner journey of healing through art. It allowed me to discover my inner being that transcended a traumatic accident and helped me overcome the unbearable loss of my eye, compounded by losing my husband to suicide.

I have heard that in order to heal, one has to undergo an altered state of consciousness. Art offers that, for it provides an avenue into a higher vibrational energetic field of consciousness, helping us to tap into other realities. In my personal journey, I experienced an altered state of consciousness through a deep contemplative state. By practicing inner and outer silence, I experienced a mystical awakening to the sacred. I felt the oneness of Love to the extent that I heard inner voices asking me questions, leading me to write a collection of psalms. Writing psalms allowed me to unleash the flow of horror and fear and praise that otherwise could not be expressed in polite company. Through my connection with the divine within, the loss of my eye resulted in my discovery of the loss of my "I," my "self," my ego, self-identity, my usual state of being, I entered into an altered state of consciousness and experienced an inner awakening to Cosmic Love, to Source for survival and ultimate surrender.

As we venture into our inner world, we capture the artist inside us. When this occurs, we awaken to healing the "hole," an empty space within controlled by the ego and the outer world of fear. Through this book, we enter the mystical unknown, a world of altered states, ritual, and ceremony. We hear within and without through words and psalms or through imagery, music, and movement. We explore sacred processes to find our self. Through the joyous wonder of our inner artist, we heal our self. This book teaches us to transcend medicine and our life's struggles, sufferings, and adventures on the physical plane. Paradoxically, we discover that embodying and grounding the inner artist is the ultimate source for healing our humanity.

—Jean Watson,
PhD, RN, AHN-BC, FAAN,
author of *Human Caring Science*

# PREFACE

Healing with arts is a powerful medicine—the most powerful that we know of to heal the whole person on physical, vital, mental, emotional, psychic, and spiritual levels. That's a big statement coming from a physician and a nurse who have worked in healthcare for most of our lives. We wrote this book because healing with arts has changed our lives and the lives of thousands of people we have had the honor to work with and teach during our sixty combined years in the Arts in Medicine field.

When we say "art" we mean *visual arts* (painting, drawing, photography, film, sculpture), *literary arts* (journaling, poetry, creative writing, theater), music (listening, playing instruments, making playlists, chanting, toning, bells, drum circles), and dance (dancing, yoga, ceremony, choreographed ritual). Arts like cooking, gardening, and decorating your house—anything that brings creativity and beauty into your life—are also included.

When we say "healing" we mean working with *physical illness, mental illness, infertility, emotional problems, life crises, grief, trauma, personal growth, family relationships, work problems, and spiritual growth*—anything that needs to be healed in your life. Healing does not always mean curing, but it can mean greatly improving your life, getting better in the broadest possible way to include your whole life.

When you put art and healing together, you get an innovative way of healing that gives you the ability to journey inward into the place of creativity. This is a mind-body state that heals on a deep physiological level.

All over the world, people are healing themselves, others, their communities, and the earth with the arts. This includes women in the Middle East painting to heal their spirits, survivors of sexual abuse, trauma, or rape dancing in the United States, veterans with post traumatic stress disorder (PTSD) painting to heal the wounds of war in Washington, DC, one woman writing and singing a song for her sick baby, and another in the Philippines painting to heal the suffering of her indigenous culture. Healing happens everywhere, from music concerts to heal the community in Newtown, Connecticut, to children with cancer dancing in hospital art and medicine programs, to women painting to heal breast cancer in San Francisco. In the next twelve weeks, we want to show you how to use art as a vehicle for healing in your own life.

Our program is different from other methods of healing or changing your life. It does not involve psychology, psychotherapy, theory, diagnosis, or treatment. It does not even involve judgment or criticism. It does not require a trained therapist, guru, or leader (although you can do the program with a therapist if you wish). You do not need to believe in any particular paradigm, religious dogma, or spiritual belief. You simply need to make art to heal, using your own innate creativity to take you inward on a personal healing journey. We have found that creativity implemented in this way is the ideal vehicle for life transformation, change, and healing, as it makes the deep healing process simple and accessible to everyone. In our art and healing method, you are the artist-healer; you learn how to do the process yourself.

The process is simple and natural. Using the imagination, we bring light to the darkness of what is blocking us or needs to be healed in our life. We see images that we can extract and bring into the light of day in the form of art that speaks from the soul. The creative process, in turn, affects our immune system, blood flow, and attitude and helps us heal. In this way, healing with art adds a new dimension to allopathic medicine, such as drugs and surgery. Art adds creativity, spirituality, love, and soul—vital elements in the health of an individual.

We know this because art has deeply healed both of us in a way that profoundly changed who we were. For Mary, it was healing her severe depression with painting. For Michael, it was working with a patient who used painting to help heal her arthritis and chronic pain. After our respective personal experiences of creating life-changing art, we each became deeply involved in the creation of the field of Arts in Medicine. Mary cofounded Shands Arts in Medicine with Dr. John Graham-Pole in Gainesville, Florida. Michael cofounded Art as a Healing Force with his sister, Linda Samuels, in Bolinas, California.

## The Dawn of Arts in Medicine

It was the early 1990s. The modern Arts in Medicine movement was gaining momentum in the United States, with hospital programs at medical centers at University of Florida, Duke University, University of Michigan, and University of Washington. These programs began by putting art on hospital walls to uplift and change the environment to a healing space, and they soon progressed. Art was brought into the interior design of hospitals, further integrating art—shapes, shades, textures, and sounds—into hospital spaces to intentionally promote healing.

The next step was the awareness that creativity could heal patients directly. This resulted in an artists-at-the-bedside initiative. Shands Arts was one of the first programs of this kind. Mary, a registered nurse, partnered with Dr. Graham-Pole, a pediatric oncologist at Shands Hospital, to start an artist-in-residence program in which artists could bring their art into the hospital in creative and innovative ways. The idea was to create opportunities for patients to integrate the arts into their lives and hardships and become involved in their own creativity, thereby finding their lights within and healing themselves. The basic assumption was that

*Everyone is an artist; everyone is a healer.*

With a small grant from the Children's Miracle Network, they bought art supplies and set up a studio space in Dr. Graham-Pole's bone marrow transplant ward where artists could meet. The first artist-in-residence was Mary's best friend, Lee Ann Stacpoole, who had helped Mary paint in her time of need when she was ill. The second artist-in-residence was Mary Lisa Katakis, a painter who also was a T-shirt artist. Then more and more artists were added.

There were endless opportunities for artists to stretch their creative talents at Shands. They could perform in the atrium, work with patients in a unit, make puppets, or implement a long-term hospital-wide art project. The most essential components involved being willing to spontaneously harness their soul's creative energy for any situation, keeping people focused on their own creativity, and seeing them and honoring them as a person, letting artist-patients articulate their own vision and dream. We found that when you believed in the artists, they believed both in themselves and in the inherent creativity of the patients and staff.

That is how Shands Arts in Medicine program was born at the University of Florida. The program currently consists of sixteen paid artists-in-residence whose work appears in five buildings of the hospital. There are musicians, visual artists, dancers, and storytellers, as well as visiting artists who play music, dance, draw and sculpt, write poetry, tell stories, and dress up as clowns. The artists give life and vibrancy to the hospital halls, drawing more people toward creativity's transformational power.

What began with volunteers has become an internationally known program, a leader in the field of arts in healthcare. Arts in Medicine humanizes the hospital and allows new healing energy and beauty to come into spaces that can be very clinical. As a result, many new programs have been created using the Shands Arts in Medicine model.

An excerpt from the film *Color My World,* produced and directed by James Babanikos in association with WUFT-TV. This moving video shows the Shands Arts in Medicine program at the University of Florida.
http://www.youtube.com/watch?v=e3CNKfJWebk&list=PLMm-0ccB
-CYpmKktLEws7WlrNyNg2QDnu&index=17

In 1991, as Mary was getting Shands Arts in Medicine off the ground and leaders of other growing Arts in Medicine programs established Society for the Arts in Healthcare in Washington, DC (now called Global Alliance for Arts and Health). The Society was a network of hundreds of professionals, students, and organizations in the arts, humanities, and medicine. The Society's mission was to explore what art and healing could mean to a hospital and its community. One of the first nonprofits involved in art and healing was Michael's organization, Art as a Healing Force, which he cofounded with his sister, an artist and museum curator, in 1989.

Art as a Healing Force was inspired by Michael's profound experience on the summit of Mount Tamalpais with visiting sculptor-healer James Surls, a Texas artist who carved spirits into his woodwork. James collected eucalyptus saplings about two inches in width and more than ten feet tall to hold a kaleidoscope of multicolored prayer flags. At the top of Tamalpais, Michael and James held on to the poles and ran down the grassy hill like soaring eagles with tree-trunk wings and colored-fabric feathers. During this run, Michael had a vision of two figures making love in free fall. They were Art and Healing, lovers combining into one. In that moment, he knew that he had to devote his life to helping make art and healing one.

Through a grant from the Rockefeller Family Fund, Michael and his sister started Art as a Healing Force. The nonprofit devoted itself to exploring how art and healing are one. They networked hospital programs, made exhibitions of healing art, and sponsored patient-care art projects with artists. They also created a slide library of thousands of artists who shared personal stories of how art had healed them, their communities, and the earth, which became the driving mission of the organization. (The library is accessible on the Arts and Healing Network's website, artheals.org.)

Art as a Healing Force worked with patients and hosted exhibitions; its annual conference at Commonweal in Bolinas, California, brought together artists, hospital program directors, philanthropists, and university professors who all examined the idea of art as a way of healing. The original participants in Art as a Healing Force conferences include many artist-healers you will meet in this book, including Vijali Hamilton, a stone sculptor who founded the World Wheel Project; Alex Grey, a visionary artist who the founded Chapel of Sacred Mirrors (CoSM); and Christiane Corbat, a visual artist who worked with women with breast cancer.

❧   ❧   ❧

More than two decades have passed since cofounding our respective programs. Today the Creative Healing field vibrates with life as a powerful force in healthcare. As the field has expanded, many more studies have been launched and hospital programs have been established. Today more than half of the major medical centers and large hospitals in the United States, as well as outpatient programs, schools, and retirement homes, have an Arts in Medicine program where patients can make art to heal.

Artists work in hospitals, programs for veterans, and community centers to heal the elderly, children, people coping with poverty, and people living with AIDS. The art-healing philosophy is taken into consideration in new and exciting ways during the development of new hospitals, where music, theater, and other arts are integrated into patient care, and visitors, families, and caregivers are also taken into consideration.

Society for the Arts in Healthcare now holds an annual conference that hundreds of artist-healers and program directors attend. Not only are there Arts in Medicine programs in most large medical centers in the United States but many programs also exist all over the world. One artist-healer works to heal people affected by the devastation of tsunamis in Japan. Others concentrate on bringing together war-torn communities; in the Middle East, an artist named JR shared on his huge Face 2 Face project to bring the Israeli and Palestinian sides together. There are massive worldwide art-healing events and movements, such as Eve Ensler's One Billion Rising and the United Nations' "One Woman" song. There is also an emerging field of environmental art that works to heal all kinds of ecosystems, from rivers and meadows to old parking lots and cityscapes, like the work of Betsy Damon, who makes art environments in China to heal water. Each day the field of Arts in Medicine grows and becomes more exciting.

This diversity of so many touching stories is a true testament to the power of art, which crosses all cultural and language barriers. We have each been witness to countless moments in which people's spirits became illuminated and were healed through the Arts in Medicine hospital programs we helped develop. We'd like to share one of these stories with you—the first of many. It's about a mother's love for her daughter and the way dancing brought them together. It is proof that art heals, that creativity applied to healthcare can help people of all types find the wholeness they're looking for.

## Maria's Story: Dancing with Angels

I am sitting on the edge of Maria's bed. We have been in the hospital off and on for many months; it feels like many years. She is so beautiful when she sleeps. I listen to her breath, her body so tiny and fragile. She gets a little smaller each day. She's my baby, and I love her more than anything.

It's been such a long and painful journey. Last year she was diagnosed with leukemia. She had all the chemotherapy, weeks and weeks of radiation, and finally a bone marrow transplant. She rallied and was clear. It was a celebration.

During those hospitalizations, Arts in Medicine played a wonderful part in her treatment. Jill, the dancer, would come in every day. She would throw ribbons around the room and dance, waving her beautiful colored scarves. Maria loved it so much. She would giggle and move and flow with the music. She always waited for the dancer to come back.

Mary Lisa, the painter, made Maria a T-shirt with her favorite kitten on it. Maria was so proud of that shirt that she wouldn't take it off for three days. We made a hat for her bald head that matched her T-shirt.

A musician visited to play Maria's favorite songs, "Twinkle, Twinkle, Little Star" and "Itsy Bitsy Spider." At the times when Maria was sickest from chemotherapy, the musician would come in and just sit on the edge of her bed and sing to her.

One day she was so sick she couldn't do anything, and the next she was better. It was a really bumpy ride. She slept more and more each day. After a long hospital stay, we went home; we went back to the cancer clinic for a follow-up. Before the doctor even came into the room, Maria looked at me with her beautiful brown saucer eyes and a sweet smile. Her hair was sparse, just growing back. She said, "Mommy, the bad cells are back." My heart sank. I knew it was over. The tests confirmed it. We thought we had made it to the other side. Now it was just a matter of time.

Back in hospital room, I just sat there. It was the last hospitalization, and no one came. The nurses couldn't look into Maria's eyes. Conversations with the residents were short. Her father stared out the window and would not talk.

The next day, there was a gentle tap on the door. It was Jill the dancer. She asked, "Is she up for dancing?"

Maria's eyes were closed, but just then she opened them and said, "Oh, yes. Yes, I want to dance." At that moment, life returned to her body.

The dancer gently lifted Maria off the bed and onto her feet, and the two started dancing together. Maria twirled and giggled, floating on the music, the silk scarves waving around her head. It was so beautiful watching my precious little girl dance. Tears rolled down my cheeks. I can still hear the soft giggles that floated around the room that day. I will hold on to that precious moment in my heart for the rest of my life.

As she danced, Maria did a perfect little twirl. Then she paused and said, "Mommy, don't worry about me. I am going to heaven and I will be dancing with the angels." She did a curtsy and another twirl. Tears fell from the dancer's eyes. Maria stood there as the most beautiful little dancer on earth.

> She climbed back into the bed, and I tucked the sheets around her. She was so happy and content. I thanked Jill for dancing. Maria passed shortly after.

We can see in Maria's story how important Arts in Medicine can be during a hospital stay; it changes everything. A beloved daughter becomes a beautiful dancer in an impossibly difficult time. The mother's final memory of her child is as an angel; what this contributed to her grieving process is beyond analysis. What it did for Maria, so close to death, seeing herself dancing with the angels, transcends understanding. Dance brought a deep spirituality and humanity to the healthcare process for Maria's family while they experienced a crisis that truly needed a healing spirit.

Time and time again, we see how using art to heal improves attitude, decreases the need for pain medication, improves communication between staff members, bonds families, and gives hope, joy, and love. Patients and staff alike become more relaxed and uplifted; they are changed and healed. Everyone is touched. No drug or treatment can do this.

Maria's story is an inspiration for us all. Creativity truly heals when it illuminates the passionate, vibrant spirit within. If it can happen in a hospital with a little girl close to death, it can happen to you. All our spirits can be illuminated with art.

## The Twelve-Week Program Is Born

After years of helping to develop Arts in Medicine and networking worldwide, and witnessing and hearing so many stories like Maria's, we realized that the illumination of the spirit could be shared beyond hospital walls. So we collaborated to create a university-level class that would teach people to become artist-healers.

Michael taught Art and Healing at San Francisco State University, in the Institute for Holistic Health Studies (IHHS), and at the John F. Kennedy University in the Master of Arts in Consciousness and Transformative Studies program. Mary taught Creativity and Spirituality in Healthcare to graduate and undergraduate students at the University of Florida. Both courses were based on our first book together, *Creative Healing*.

As we taught, we realized that the students experienced major healing that was as profound as our patients' transformations. Time and time again, student course evaluations and papers went beyond expectations in writing about illuminating their spirits, helping with grief, and healing depression, sexual abuse, and illness. They wrote of major life changes, changing careers, improving family, switching life direction, feeling more at peace, and finding who they were as people. They experienced themselves in lucid and enlightened ways, with the full wholeness of being alive. One day, as we read the evaluations and told each other the moving and exciting stories of projects students had done in each of our classes, we realized that we needed to write a book. We understood that we had created a twelve-week program for profound life change and healing using art. We had developed a healing method that produced real life change that needed to be shared. We have taken Art and Healing out of the hospital and give it to you so that you can heal yourself, others, or the earth.

This book is an invitation for you to experience creative healing. We are honored to share our commitment, experiences, and skills to create a personal journey for you to experience art as a healing force. We hope this book will serve as a dear friend, guide, and teacher. We support, honor, and encourage you. This book calls for you to heal—because as you heal yourself, you are ultimately healing all of humanity. Your life is your unique gift to everyone. To heal loved ones, your community, or the world, you must begin by healing yourself.

# INTRODUCTION

*We are at a breaking point in medicine where . . . arts, spirituality, and healing . . . are coming together to produce a new multidimensional model for healthcare. Now arts interventional modalities are as powerful as clinical medical interventions.*

**—Leland Kaiser,** health futurist and associate professor
in Health Administration, University of Colorado, at Denver

The basic premise of using art to heal is simple: each of us has an inner artist and an inner healer. The inner artist is the part of you that is passionately creative, falls in love, feels connected to everything around you, can see and make things, is at home with yourself, and is willing to explore. The inner healer is the part that balances your body, keeps you alive and growing, and, most important, heals you. It is the part of you that regulates the self-healing mechanisms that cure infection, cancer, and other illnesses.

Using art as a healing force essentially frees the inner healer by embracing the passionate, creative artist in each of us. You can use art to heal yourself, others, some aspect of your community, or the earth—all by tapping into the creative energy that makes you alive.

The first goal of this twelve-week program is to help you marry your inner artist with your inner healer to change your body's physiology through the creative process, thereby optimizing healing and renewal. By releasing tension and fear and opening the mind to passionate creativity and the forces that created us, the inner artist and healer merge as one. They release the immense energetic power of love to attain balanced wholeness. It's the oldest healing known and is now recognized as the most advanced by health futurists.

The greatest healer in your life resides within you. Listen to the teachings and wisdom from inside. Slow down enough to tap into your creative forces. Your destiny is to become fully alive, free, and aware of yourself. Our goal is to bring out your creativity and integrate it as part of your healing, using the same process we teach in the hospitals and in our university classes. Treat this book as a creative tool during your journey.

This experience is intended to be exciting and joyful. Make it fun; it's an adventure, a time to remember and return to what you love and are most passionate about.

## The Research Behind This Book

When Mary completed her PhD thesis at the University of Florida College of Nursing, she published a peer-reviewed medical research study in the journal *Cancer Nursing* that showed how art healed by illuminating spirit. Our previous book, *Spirit Body Healing*, told the stories of the people in Mary's study. From her research, we developed the Spirit Body Healing method, which is now used with cancer patients and people with illness and life crises. This method plays a large role in the twelve-week course we are about to embark on together; you'll be able to use its eight themes throughout your own process.

In the study, Mary interviewed people who had healed themselves with art—patients and families in a hospital setting who had worked with Shands Arts in Medicine, artists, and visionary artist-healers. Mary interviewed or visited each person in their studio, where they shared art, poetry, and videos. These people answered the question, "What was your own experience of making art to heal?"

Mary conducted detailed interviews of people who had been through life crises or healed themselves of life-threatening illness. She analyzed their stories to elucidate the themes of how personal healing occurred. Mary's study revealed more than questions on a questionnaire, which are sometimes narrow and only ask what the researcher already knew. With this kind of qualitative health research—known as hermeneutic phenomenology—Mary used real-life stories, photographs, and art as data to inform her research about the complex process behind creative healing.

Although the project took more than four years, Mary got answers that were powerful, surprising, and beyond expectations. In her final analysis, she made a major discovery from the patterns that emerged from the interviews. What people said over and over again was that they went to a place inside themselves where they experienced a shift of consciousness. This allowed them to see their whole life in a new way. When the change in perspective occurred, the life healing began. Although the experiences were different for each person, the underlying theme was the same. Each person went from a place of profound darkness, fear, or illness to a place where they experienced luminous transcendence. People described feeling intensely alive and transformed. From the metamorphosis, their spirit became palpably awakened and illuminated. The answer was that art heals by facilitating a spiritual experience that is deep and beautiful.

The Spirit Body Healing method comes from peer-reviewed research on real patients in a hospital setting. The method's eight themes come from ordinary people—patients with stories of pain and suffering who chose to live their lives in extraordinary ways.

## The Eight Themes of How Art Heals

In evaluating the data from the research, Mary found eight simple themes that emerged from participant interviews, giving us a road map of the process of healing with art. The themes are a solid framework you can use throughout the art and healing process. As you make art to heal, you can see where you are on the road map the themes provide and understand more deeply what is happening to you. You are not alone; the exciting transformation process you are undergoing is one that many people before you have experienced as well.

1. Pain and Darkness
2. Going Elsewhere
3. Art as a Turning Point
4. Slipping Through the Veil
5. Trusting the Process
6. Embodying Spirit
7. Feeling the Healing Energy of Love and Compassion
8. Experiencing Transcendence

Of course, the journey you take through these themes may not go in this particular order. The order is often mixed; sometimes multiple themes happen at once. Some people don't go through all the themes. Some people go right to Experiencing Transcendence without spending much time in Pain and Darkness. Regardless, the process is simple for everyone. It will naturally come to you.

As you undertake the twelve-week process, you'll be able see which theme you are working on. Think about how the themes apply to your life and to the creative work you will be doing. As you read stories of people's experiences, you'll see examples of the themes as they move from darkness to transcendence.

## Theme One: Pain and Darkness

Where did the stories begin? First, each person interviewed shared a story of pain and darkness, a moment when they were afraid, in pain, suffering, or crisis. Their examples included physical pain, a new cancer diagnosis, divorce, personal crisis, or loss. Many stories started in fear or with a hurtful, life-threatening event. In each case, healing started with a darkness that needed to be changed.

In every story, the people who healed themselves and changed their lives started by realizing that their pain and darkness was something that needed to be healed by going *toward* this pain and darkness. People who are ill suffer. People in life crises suffer. Going into your pain and darkness—facing it, bringing it out—is crucial to stopping the suffering. The steps to dealing with pain and darkness are facing the pain, characterizing and describing it, bringing it outside you, and doing something creative with it.

We should mention that for the creative healing process, not everyone starts in personal darkness. Many people don't need to heal themselves; they choose to heal others, their community, or the earth. The darkness for them is not personal but communal. The darkness can be illness in another person, violence toward women, problems experienced by the elderly or a minority group, or even environmental issues like air and water quality.

## Theme Two: Going Elsewhere

Facing pain and darkness takes people "elsewhere." As you extract the pain, you bring yourself to a place where you can see yourself from a more objective perspective. This place is not the place where you are in pain; it is elsewhere. In making art, the experience of making art with the intention to heal can also transport you elsewhere. Your first piece of art is a journey away from the pain to a new place. The art itself is the elsewhere. A woman in the Arts in Medicine program who was sexually abused told us that when she painted the picture of her spirit animal, she left the darkness. She spent time with her magic healing creature, which protected her from harm. She was elsewhere, bathed in light, not alone in the darkness anymore.

### Theme Three: Art as a Turning Point

Next, participants become immersed in their creative process. Whether it's making art, painting, sculpting, dancing, journal writing, composing poetry, tending a garden, or going on a trip, art becomes an all-encompassing activity that changes their lives. Some people make hundreds of pieces of art to heal. Their work goes on for years, becoming a lifelong activity.

### Theme Four: Slipping through the Veil

After you allow yourself to be taken into the pain, go elsewhere, and make art, you meet with your own spirit. The spirit moves from the deepest part within you into your outer life. The spirit connects with you. You are taken within the darkness and pain, but you realize you are not alone. There is something greater than you—a spirit you become connected to. In one interviewee's words, "you slip through the veil." Suddenly you are within your own body in a place of spaciousness. One person had a dream of God; another, Jesus. Still another saw Buddha and yet another, the Universal Creator. Many people felt an experience of enlightenment. Slipping through the veil is the place of opening where people see angels; sense the presence of God or saints; and talk with grandparents, ancient ancestors, or even children who've passed away. Slipping through the veil is the result of going inward.

### Theme Five: Trusting the Process

This was a wonderful experience for many people in the research study. It was like coming home. They understood that making art was their vehicle for healing. Acceptance turned into self-knowledge. In this stage, you become a witness of your own life. You know you have found the truth. You now are on the path of greater good, and you exist for the greater good of others. You create a place where you have faith because of your own experience of being embraced by an infinite love. Every moment is precious. Every moment is being with spirit in a spiritual dimension.

Knowing the truth is an experience, not a theory. It is a powerful feeling of correctness, liberation, being at home at last, and understanding what has been puzzling you. Knowing the truth is a feeling of certainty, well-being, and harmony with the universe.

Knowing the truth about who you are and your purpose helps you make harmonious decisions in your life.

In this step, people describe how the process of Spirit Body Healing feels. They often said it was similar to moving like a river and that they would "keep flowing." As they saw themselves moving and flowing, they would see themselves change. Some people describe this process as "being with the next breath." Others told Mary that it was about being present and allowing the process to define them. Surrendering involved releasing the Inner Critic and letting go of criticism, judgment, or self-condemnation. In surrender, a person allows fear and inadequacies to exist. They accept emotions, including pain, despair, and rage. Surrender also involves expressing these feelings. It includes allowing the storms and hurricanes to be, accepting the velocity of energy that gets released in life. Surrender is about accepting your own darkness and accepting yourself as a conduit for your emotions.

Surrender is also about focusing on your emotions. You make a decision and bring intention to the focusing itself. You may concentrate on despair, embody the pain, become one with it, and merge with it. Surrender is an emotional and physical sensation, a letting go that reveals who you are.

## Theme Six: Embodying Spirit

After the knowing of the truth, you enter a beautiful and radiant experience. These new images often show you that you are strong, beautiful, powerful, or healed. In Mary's research, the person often felt reborn as a brand-new person. In enchantment and embodiment of spirit, a person's senses are awakened. Their body is connected to spirit. People said that they knew what this is for the first time. Sounds became more intense. The whole body and its senses were more sensitive. People felt their vitality and recognized it in others—"the experience of being truly alive." People said that they were alive in the world for the first time and that their lives are a wondrous gift. They felt a vortex of energy around them.

## Theme Seven: Feeling the Healing Energy of Love and Compassion

The Spirit Body Healing research showed that when the spirit was heard and seen and images of light and beauty emerged, the person would have enormous feelings of healing. There were physical sensations of energy, buzzing, vibration, calmness, pleasant sensations, and joy. Participants described this state as being within a "vortex of energy," feeling excited, exhilarated, fully alive. These feelings were not asked for or expected; the person did not have to do anything to get them. The experience was always concrete and unmistakable. In this enchanted state, ecstasy and energy are not theoretical things or metaphysical speculation; they are a unique experience shared by ordinary people healing themselves. The enchantment was different depending on the situation. If people were depressed, they would feel interest and enthusiasm; if they were ill, they would feel strength.

Mary's research showed that healing through the creative process releases the life force. When a person heals with the spirit, they understand why the Hindu religion says that energy and matter are related to consciousness.

From this, we learned that art and healing create feelings of compassion for yourself, which is crucial in the healing process. One patient told Mary that "I became compassionate by seeing myself from a distance, from outside. I stood back and said objectively, 'Look at her; she needs.'" In a moment of witness, of reflection, participants could see what they needed to heal. When you observe yourself with compassion, you can tend to yourself as a sacred body. Your emotions are natural forces that move though you. You can honor intuitions and insights. You can be illuminated and find your place in the world.

## Theme Eight: Experiencing Transcendence

In the research study, each of the people Mary talked to had profound experiences of transcendence. They experienced intense feelings of oneness and interconnectedness. These feelings were like the ones they'd had in slipping through the veil, but now the feelings were deeper, more fully formed and experienced. Earlier glimpses of God angels or other spirits grew in clarity. They often experienced the power of the universe or God and even heard the voice of God. They felt they had emerged in another dimension of great power and beauty. People felt like they were a vehicle to share and communicate love from a place of constant renewable ecstasy. One woman told us,

I spent years trying to find myself. I did it all. I tried body work, meditation, Rolfing, and women's groups. Then I got really sick. I went inside myself and painted. Then I found myself, right smack inside. It's the biggest joke in the world. You go out in the world to find yourself and find her inside. Who would have thought?

All the subjects described experiences of becoming filled with power or light. They described seeing aspects of themselves they had never known. Their senses had become illuminated and clear. They described feeling like they could see deeply or hear intensely for the first time. They told stories of joy, gratitude, and celebration. They realized that their bodies are divine.

This was the most important finding of the study and the reason Mary called her research study Spirit Body Healing. After a person goes inward, glimpses darkness, sees the light, and feels the energy of their spirit, they heal. Each person had a different experience of transcendence, but it was a recognizable and repeatable phenomenon.

## How to Use This Book

Everyone can use this program, whether your intention is to heal yourself, practice with an artist-healer, or work with a trained art therapist. If you already consider yourself an artist or healer, we'll show you how to go deeper into your creativity. You can heal emotionally, intellectually, and spiritually. Your mind will show you how the art and healing worlds are naturally linked; the artist can be the voice and hands of the healer within.

There are twelve chapters in this book, which represent the twelve weeks of the Art as a Healing Force course. In our experience, we've found that this life transformation is most effective when completed in twelve weeks over a three-month period. It generally takes people three months to commit time to empowering themselves. In these three months, we make the space and complete the process of growing and creating deeper meaning in our lives. This includes changing your lifestyle, accomplishing new goals, executing a plan of action, or inspiring yourself to start a lifelong creative healing process. This program can be done over a shorter or longer period of time to fit your own schedule and needs as well. Each week can be stretched out, for example; or you can jump between some weeks in parts 2 and 3, depending on your preference—just as long as you complete part 1. Ultimately, the twelve weeks are just the beginning of the process; art and healing is life work. Once you start, you won't be able to go back to the noncreative healing life.

### *Weekly Schedule*

Each of the three parts in this book is made up of four chapters, one per week. Each week is broken into two main sections.

1. *Weekly lesson:* The first part of the chapter introduces the week's theme and provides the necessary information and research so you can understand how the material applies directly to change in your own life. We also include stories about some of the participants in our classes as well as artist-healer profiles of pioneers in the field.

2. *Weekly praxis:* The word *praxis* comes from the ancient Greek for "a practical action for a goal." Praxis is the process through which a skill is enacted, embodied, and realized. As Picasso said, "Inspiration exists, but it has to find you working." Transformation takes more than reading a book; it is about commitment and taking action. For this journey, you must fully participate in healing your own life. The second part of the chapter contains the hands-on art-healing praxis. It starts with guided imagery exercises that will lead you into your visionary world. Then it gives instructions for how to make healing art so that you can experience the phenomenon for yourself.

At the end of each week, there is a summary of the guided imagery and Medicine Art for the week so you can quickly refer back to what you need to accomplish. We also list additional art projects at the end of each week.

## A Call to Healing

In the style of our university classes, we begin each week with a call to healing. This invokes a supportive, caring environment that honors your creative healing process and helps you get in the art-healing mind-set going into the chapter. It's a simple weekly ceremony you can also perform before you begin working creatively. This is a great ceremony for an art-healing group, too, as it gets everyone on the same wavelength.

## Guided Imagery

Guided imagery is a big part of the praxis section. Like riding a bicycle, it may seem foreign at first, especially if you've never tried it. However, it's easy to start cruising artistically with this powerful tool for the imagination.

We are both recognized experts in guided imagery. We have used guided imagery with students and patients on a day-to-day basis for many years. Michael wrote the first major book on guided imagery in 1975, the bestselling *Seeing with the Mind's Eye*, and Mary teaches guided imagery with the renowned Jean Watson to train nurses at the Watson Caring Science Institute. Guided imagery is a goal of our art and healing process. Once you learn it and are comfortable with it, it's a life skill you can use in daily life and sports and in healing and relaxation. It's fun, exciting, surprising, moving, and healing. It offers something completely new for everyone.

Guided imagery gives you an immediate experience of your visionary world as well as imagery to make art. This visual imagery also has an impact on your physiology. Your experience of imagery, whether through sight, sound, or mental imagery, is a body experience, too. The image you hold in your brain does not have to be real or even exist. All that's important is that you see it in your mind's eye and imagine it clearly. For example, if you see a stick in the road and you think it's a snake, you go into the fight or flight response—your heart speeds up, your breathing accelerates, blood flow to your digestive organs slows, and blood to your big muscles increases, even though it is only a piece of wood. In a similar way, if you imagine a healing scene, you don't have to be there. Your body will react as if it's there and go into healing physiology. When you picture a scene that is beautiful and moving, your body reacts with joy and relaxation. We'll be discussing this phenomenon more in the weeks ahead.

## *Medicine Art*

Medicine Art is another vital aspect of your weekly praxis. When you make art with the intent to heal, you make art as medicine. The intent to make art to heal is healing, as is the creative process. Art truly becomes your medicine. Your Medicine Art has healing power. Indigenous peoples called the sacred art objects they made to heal "medicine" because it held healing energy. Medicine for these people surpassed drugs and surgery. It meant deep healing. Medicine Art has vibrational energy because it is your dream of healing projected outward and made manifest in the world.

All Medicine Art helps you harness your creative power. Your medicine taps into your own life experience. Your huge creative energy allows you to gain confidence and see your own truth, wisdom, and spirit. You will be able to reveal and proudly show yourself to those around you. From our experience in the art and healing field, this creates deep healing as well as personal revelations.

Our first Medicine Art project starts in week 1. In the book, we've kept each week's core Medicine Art project relatively simple. You will draw from the images and emotional content that arise during the guided imagery tours. Those who want to learn about more Medicine Art can visit this book's website, healingwiththearts.com.

## *Journaling*

Every guided imagery and Medicine Art activity will involve journaling. In our twelve-week process, the journal documents your creative process as it evolves. The journal captures all your ideas in one place. You may write what you see in your guided imagery, for example. It is also a wonderful place to draw, sketch, write, and paste. Refer back to it. Simple journaling has been shown to have incredible health benefits because it

- Decreases the number of illness episodes
- Promotes sleep
- Enhances immune function
- Reduces alcohol consumption
- Increases communication, socialization, and connection with others when you write about traumatic events and emotions
- Increases re-evaluation and understanding of life circumstances
- Supports self-reflection
- Helps identify interpersonal and environmental triggers
- Tracks anxiety-producing emotions and feelings or symptoms of illness
- Records patterns of pain and pain management
- Translates inchoate emotions and emotional experiences into words

In our university classes, the journal has become a vital tool of self-discovery for our students, and we promise it will be that for your journey as well. Your journal will get full and used. And if our past art-healing students' and patients' experiences are any indication, it will be personal, colorful, and rich.

### *Art-Healing Stories and Artist-Healer Profiles*

We can tell you from experience that your Medicine Art will be completely different from the projects you read about here. To help you identify what needs to be healed, we have included special sections throughout the chapters designed to share how other class participants and patients have used art to heal themselves. These intimate true stories of how people healed with our twelve-week process or in the clinical setting are examples of what people can do. These stories will help you understand what is happening in your body.

To help provide some further inspiration, we also introduce artist-healer profiles in parts 2 and 3. You'll meet some of the world's leading artist-healers, and you'll see how many ways artists are using their creativity to heal themselves, others, and the world.

### *Media Tags*

Finally, throughout the book, we've provided specially coded tags you can scan with your smartphone to access more content on our website, including videos, images, and more. Be on the lookout for these as you read.

### *Final Project*

The whole point of these guided imagery exercises and Medicine Art projects is to help you explore yourself. The work will prepare you for your final Medicine Art project, the pinnacle of the twelve-week process. Every class participant creates a project at the end of the program. Keep this final project in mind through the whole program.

Whether you want to heal a physical illness, psychological problem, or emotional issue or you aspire to achieve personal growth, know that the people who have done the process have made the most exciting and moving projects imaginable. No one could have dreamed of what they'd do when they started. They have healed lifelong back pain; healed from sexual abuse and rape; relieved side effects of cancer treatments; and healed from many physical and mental illnesses with painting, fabric arts, dance, and music. They have grieved the death of family members and broken relationships. They have built benches in their homes for peace, written poetry for a brother who was ill, painted their Inner Critic away, and made huge goddesses to heal their divine feminine.

They have healed babies and families in neonatal care units with poetry, healed elders in assisted care facilities with music, and helped their grandfather with Alzheimer's disease with music. They have healed rivers by cleaning up garbage, healed mountains with huge sculptures, and even healed communities from violence with large dance ceremonies. Thousands of different projects have been completed. Each time, they surprise the artists and us as well. They are more than we'd ever dreamed they could be and are truly life changing.

Each week's guided imagery and Medicine Art will guide you through this transformative process, step by step. You will begin by finding something in your life that needs healing, then an art media to use, and then a process to use the art. Each chapter will have examples of projects and exercises to help each step. At the end of the twelve-week process, we will have a graduation ceremony. This ceremony of initiation as a healing artist will complete your work and help you begin a new life as an artist-healer. From there, you can go anywhere and do anything. We'll be focusing much more on the final Medicine Art project starting in week 4.

## Forming an Art-Healing Group

If you complete this twelve-week process on your own, it will be a powerful life-changing experience. You can also complete this process with other people in an intentional healing, caring community. This book, after all, was born from our university classes, which themselves originated from Arts in Medicine programs that focus so intently on the healing effects of a loving, supportive, familial community.

When we teach our courses at the University of Florida, John F. Kennedy University, and San Francisco State University, we usually assemble a group of about twenty to forty people for the class. Because the curriculum focuses on art and healing, about half our groups are in art—graduate students in ceramics, film, music, painting—and the other half are in healing—nurses, premedical students, physical therapists, psychologists. They can be any age from twenty to seventy years old with a wide range of backgrounds and lifestyles. Since ceramic artists don't really end up hanging out with nurses at the university, they usually don't know each other and may have never seen each other before. The process is new for all of them.

In our courses, we create a caring community as a sacred space to optimize the art and healing experience. This community is intentionally created and crafted to be loving and nonjudgmental. We establish this kind of communal environment from the first day of the process. Being in community and sharing is just as important for some people as making art. Part of healing is being who you are authentically, allowing yourself to be seen, trusted, and honored for who you are.

Since this is a book, not a class, you will need to build your caring community yourself to accompany you on this healing journey. In some ways, it's a bit easier for those at home not taking this course with a group of complete strangers; you can choose your art-healing group from your family members and friends. You can meet weekly in a home, studio, church, or community center. You can find people who want to meet once a week to share projects and stories. You can work with people in a spiritual or art community. You can also easily create an online group. Once you have completed the art-healing process, you could even facilitate a workshop yourself and teach the course.

This book is designed for both individual and group use. If you choose not to start an art-healing community, keeping a journal or documenting your process is essential. The blank page will provide a place to bounce ideas and explore your process. If you want to have cheerleaders on the sidelines—like a spouse, friend, grandmother, or people you've made art with—go for it.

## *Summary*

The twelve-week process is really simple. You complete a guided imagery each week and then you make your art from what you saw. The instructions are summarized at the end of each week's chapter.

- For each of the twelve weeks, read the chapter-opening teachings, which not only introduce the theme of each week but also describe the art-healing process through past participants' eyes to give you a better idea of what the experience can be like. Highlighted profiles of professional artist-healers are interwoven in the chapters so that you know what the week is about and can draw from the wisdom of these people.

- From the praxis, do the guided imagery of the week and then make Medicine Art from what you saw and experienced. On this book's website, we also give some alternative Medicine Art projects of the week you can try as well as embedded tags you can use to go online, get more content, and learn more.

• The guided imagery and art projects are basic to the process and will take about thirty to sixty minutes each week. The journal will take another thirty minutes. Many people get so excited when writing that they spend much more time than this.

• Think about and work on your final Medicine Art project throughout the twelve-week process. We find it best to first think, see, and plan, and then do some actual work during the middle weeks—writing and sketching in your journal, for example—and finish in the last weeks.

Of course, you can work at your own pace, which means that if the twelve-week structure doesn't fit your schedule, that's perfectly fine. Just make sure you read through all the material and focus on making this process rich, life-changing, and deeply healing.

• The teaching gives you the basic knowledge.
• The guided imagery helps you find healing images.
• The Medicine Art lets you feel, experience, and make visible and tangible the vision you drew from the guided imagery.
• Once inspired and inspirited, the art process brings the inner artist and inner healer together to create lasting change on neurological and physiological levels.

The whole process is new and at the same time ancient. The main idea is for this work to be easy and fun and to carry you up as you take a transformative journey.

From our many years of doing this program, we know that you can do this—anyone can. Creativity is in our genes; we do it naturally. We are hardwired to be creative and to use our imagination to heal, so it is the easiest, most natural process for life change. You do not need to be an artist or a healer. You just need to be human and want to heal something in your life or grow as a person.

Like any journey, it takes work and play. You can do it by yourself or with a circle of friends in your own community. We have designed this book to fit all occasions. You can work with a therapist or an art therapist. People who are art therapists, teachers, or educators can also use this book as a resource for their patients and for themselves. This book is meant to be a guidebook, companion, and support network all rolled into one so that you can facilitate your own personal healing journey. We are here with you every step of the way to support you in this exciting life-changing process. We know you can do it. Each week is a step in your healing journey of mind, body, and spirit.

This transformation will allow you to enjoy the gift of who you are as a human being. You can be authentically present and create a field of love that heals you and all the people around you. Healing with art is so potent and effective that all you have to do is follow the steps.

# PART I

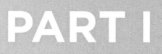

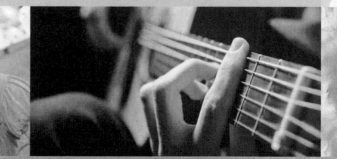

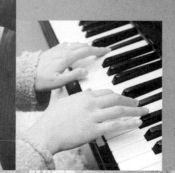

# BEGINNING *THE* JOURNEY

# Beginning the Journey

In the first four weeks of our journey, we'll show you how art lived through the heart, senses, and soul can become a vehicle of profound change and healing.

The healing art you'll produce in weeks 1 and 2 is designed to activate and unite the artist and healer within and then marry the two into one. In weeks 3 and 4, with a solid grasp of art-healing basics, we'll take the process deeper. We'll turn inward and look at what needs to be healed on your own mental, physical, or spiritual planes. By the end of part 1, you'll be a fledgling artist-healer, ready to launch into the more advanced levels of using art to heal as you approach your final Medicine Art project.

# WEEK 1

# ACTIVATING THE ARTIST
# AND HEALER WITHIN

*This is the ever-present moment to invoke the artist within.*
*The blessing of this moment is that when our hearts open, we can see*
*who we truly are, for the eye in the heart is the eye of the spirit.*

Welcome to the first week of your own Art as a Healing Force program. Whether you've formed an art-healing group or are doing this in a community of one, this week is the beginning of a very personal journey toward healing with the arts. This week we will make our first piece of healing art together.

Do not worry about whether you consider yourself an artist or a healer—trust us, you are both. We have guided thousands of people through the art-healing process over the years; anyone who has misgivings soon finds out that it's really quite easy and fun. The powerful effect of this work is that whatever adversity or hurdle people have overcome, they find a creative outlet to express their core selves and use their creative catharsis as a means for healing themselves, others, and their environment in profound ways. As Julia Cameron wrote in *The Artist's Way*, "Art opens the closets, airs out the cellars and attics. It brings healing."[1]

---

1. Julia Cameron, *The Artist's Way: A Spiritual Path to Higher Creativity* (New York: Jeremy P. Thatcher/ Putnam, 2002), 68.

Our main goal for this first week's praxis is for you to be able to locate the joyful place within you and confidently say, "I am an artist." This is the first step—re-embracing the artistry we all have within us. That's the lesson Mary had to learn before founding Shands Arts in Medicine. It was a time in her life when she had to figure out how to rediscover her passions, heal herself, and help launch an art-healing movement.

## Mary's Story: Painting to Heal

Twenty years ago, life challenged me. I became depressed, and everything in my life shattered and changed. I felt like I was drifting away from myself and all that I knew. In that moment of despair, I realized I had a vision and a dream I had never actualized. I'd always wanted to be an artist but did not have the time or skill, and did not know how to go about learning how to be one. It was a turning point in my life. I became increasingly depressed and immobilized. In spite of therapy, self-help books, and workshops, I was floundering. I was trying to find something outside myself to ease my pain.

Then there was a miracle. A friend invited me to a studio to make art. It was a ray of hope—something that interested me. Everything in my life had turned bland until I started to paint. Art became my sun, my water, and my food. It energized me so much that I felt alive again. I fell in love with becoming an artist. I started painting every day. My creative process was like a river, a wellspring of energy that was profoundly healing and transformative. This experience changed me to my core. I had an experience of healing so profound that I became well and became a different person.

I tapped into my own enthusiasm and power to experience being truly alive. I worked every day in my studio. I invited the artist into my life, and I became the artist of my own life. It was a point of departure where I never looked back. My life was on a path to fill a destiny that was unfolding. I knew something was happening that was deeply profound and connected me to my spiritual purpose.

I took out a large canvas but did not even know how to hold a brush. I looked though magazines and saw a picture of a woman who was broken and distorted. That was how I felt. I started painting. I got excited about the colors of the paint, how the shapes appeared on the paper. My painting was large. As I worked, it started to look like something—it looked like my pain, how I felt. I forgot about how I felt and instead *looked* at how I felt. I got excited about the making of the painting.

Then I got another canvas and started a series of paintings of women. They were all distorted in the beginning. I painted garish backgrounds. I took photographs of myself and started painting self-portraits. I become absorbed in the process and painted how I felt instead of thinking about how I felt. I began to realize that I was painting my life.

Next I created a studio space for myself and simply began painting. In the beginning, I made no attempt to define myself or my process. I painted from pure feeling states. I became absorbed in the pure expression and gesture of painting. I could completely release my energy passionately on the canvas. The series turned out to be self-portraits. The first painting I called *Cut Out My Heart*. It was my pain—a deeply intense and dying pain. The figure was broken, distorted, diffuse, crumpled, crying, and bleeding. I painted "her." This figure had been my despair, my uncensored and purely emotional energy. In the moment I had released this image, I stepped back, looked, and gasped. What I saw was an aspect of myself that I hadn't faced until then. It was so ugly. Yet I felt calm and detached in this moment face-to-face with myself. I had let go on an intense emotional and physical level. Painting is physical for me; I embody my pain as I paint it.

For the first time, I was experiencing my pain in a strange new way. As a painter, I stood in front of my canvas and was in control for the first time. I painted my emotions. I painted my body. I could feel that I was the creator of myself.

When I returned to my studio later, I saw that the painting had captured and contained a moment that was now in the past. The painting remained, though the emotion had passed. It was an object that contained an image created in genuine expression. I had moved past it. I realized that I was witnessing my own transformation.

As I painted a series of self-portraits, I struggled with form and perspective. Metaphorically I was re-creating and reconstructing my inner form and inner perspective. The external creative process mirrored my inner world. I realized that the manifestation of movement and change was powerful. It was a process of knowing myself. As I immersed myself in painting, I not only became well but also became the artist I had always wanted to be. My creativity was a part of myself I had neither acknowledged nor honored. Through this experience, I realized that art could be used as a vehicle for healing.

Art became a way to know myself through the experience of my pain. In seeing my emotions, I could step away from them. They became my art—completely separate from me. In essence, I became free.

I spent two years as an artist in my studio. I painted my children playing on the beach. I painted the surrounding landscapes I saw. I set up still lifes on the kitchen table to paint the things I loved.

Since I was a nurse and art had healed me, I hoped to bring art into the healthcare system. This was my opportunity to help others help themselves. No one had ever told me I could take my illness and use it constructively to help myself. Everywhere I looked it seemed like I had been in relationship with a form of healing that was disjointed from my life. It did not support me in the way I needed it to. It wasn't until I threw myself into my creative work that I felt a powerful healing effect. I needed to throw my whole life into something powerful. I needed my whole life immersed in it because that was how I was involved with my sickness. Art and healing transformed my life. I healed myself. My process was not fragmented—one hour, twice a week. My illness was so overwhelming that I needed to live my healing all the time, not just in visits to a therapist. What was going to heal me—and others—was a relationship with myself that was fundamentally different than any I had had before. I could always be there for myself.

 Mary describes how she healed herself from depression through painting. http://www.youtube.com/watch?v=PTlEj6LaPYM&list=PLMm-0ccB -CYpmKktLEws7WlrNyNg2QDnu&index=16

## Becoming an Artist-in-Residence in Life

*I realized I have an artistic side. It was a real awakening in my life.*
—**Brenda**, San Francisco State University
Institute for Holistic Health Studies

Perhaps you're thinking, "I haven't had an art project since high school," or, "No one has ever told me my art was any good." Maybe you have even been told that your art was bad. While it might be true that you haven't practiced any art for a while, the other truth is that you have been an artist since you were a child and your imaginative lightbulb was burning bright as you became the creative, capable adult you are today. Creativity is what makes us human. Though you may not have seen this or valued it, you'll be able to do so now. Embracing your inner artist is one of the most important shifts you can make in life. This is a basic foundation to using art as a healing force.

The definition of the word *artist* is much broader than most of us think. When we think "artist," we usually think of a painter, musician, dancer, or poet. But in everything you do, there are opportunities to be creative. We want to broaden our definition of art to include all aspects of life. Art is a way of being, of seeing life through a creative lens and molding our realities to fit our unique vision of the world. An artist looks deeply into each moment—the play between light and shadows, the beauty of children laughing and playing, the almost electric presence of someone you care about. When you reclaim your inner artist, an aspect of yourself is illuminated. It is a shift of who you think you are. We're all artists-in-residence in general life.

The risk of not making art is worse than the risk of making art that heals.

So, heading into the coming weeks, do not to judge yourself or the art that comes out of this process. Open yourself to your creative flow. It's not about the product but the process. This art is not to sell, nor is it a competition. It is art made intentionally to heal and truly let go.

Creatively focused healing means opening, transforming, becoming, and emerging. It means shining the light of your mind to the outside world, making the creative process a path to illumination, the spiritual glow that illuminates us when we create. Perhaps you've seen that halo-like glow surrounding people who create something that resonates with their souls. At its core, art is the expression of the spirit, the Divine Creator. No matter what your spiritual beliefs are, art heals via this creative life force. The spirit that propels us has the power to heal at the deepest level of our being. When we embody the artist within, we tap into the flow of this essential life force.

In this way, art is the portal that shares this light. Others can witness and experience the beauty within you. This light shines brightly in each human. We touch each other with artistic expressions and gifts. This kind of creativity is natural and beautiful—and healing.

### Artist-Healer Profile: Inna Dagman—
### From Dancing to Heal to Dancer-in-Residence

"When I started the Art as a Healing Force process, I did not know anything about creativity and healing. However, it changed my life. I had no idea that this project would become a portal for my own personal transformation and a reunification with my inner artist-healer core," said Inna Dagman, student at the San Francisco State University Institute for Holistic Health Studies (IHHS), who found more than just healing with art and a new way of seeing the world when she found a career in Arts in Medicine.

Inna is tall and statuesque. She looks like a dancer and has the attractiveness that comes from a good heart. Watching her make art to heal, you could see that part of her was put down by criticism and that she was disappointed with herself about certain choices she'd made in life, but you could also see her waking up to a depth she had forgotten she still had.

My path as a dancer-healer began when I did the Art as a Healing Force process. I loved dancing from a young age and took different dance classes throughout my life. However, due to my strong inclination to help others heal, I thought that my future was in the helping professions and never considered dance as a future career. Moreover, many of the dance classes I took had a highly competitive element to them. Many times I got the message that I wasn't good enough because I didn't have several years of rigorous training in ballet. More often than not, I was not getting the free-flowing creative expression my body craved in these dance classes, and I became quite disillusioned.

I was then an undergraduate student pursuing a BA in psychology. I was also working as a restaurant server. My life was consumed by school and work. I craved dance but never had the time for it. As far as I knew and heard from anyone, this was the time to sacrifice *unnecessary* things such as creative expression and focus on studying and paying bills. Although I couldn't comprehend it at the time, this existence, without any creative outlet for the soul, was deeply unfulfilling and numbing.

However, some inner part of me was crying for something else, for a deep healing and authentic expression. That is how I found myself in the Art and Healing class with Michael Samuels. The first day of class, I watched *Color My World*, the deeply moving documentary about the Shands Arts in Medicine program. When I saw Jill Sonke dancing at patients' bedsides, I knew it was something I would love to do. I knew I could do it naturally. Dance was flowing with a healing intention and filling the hospital room with light. This was very different from what I had experienced in my dance classes, which left me feeling bad about myself and my ability. I was very deeply touched, and I was scared because I wasn't ready to change my whole life and path.

Inna was like a lot of people who first entered the program; she did not know about art and healing but knew that something inside her called her to explore the unknown. She still had an inkling of passion burning for dance but never dreamed that she'd do it in any mature, meaningful capacity. The Art as Healing Force program's open, supportive environment nurtured parts of Inna that came to light with each drawing, poem, and movement of her sacred, beautiful dance.

"The dance movements seemed to flow out of a deep place within me," Inna told us. "They came from a place of no judgment—of complete acceptance and love—a place of healing energy."

We will be following Inna's story and others from the Art as a Healing Force class as the weeks progress, and we will learn more about these students' experiences, impressions, and art to demonstrate the diverse avenues healing can take.

## The Muse That Heals

As these stories attest, when art is expressed from the deepest levels of our being, profound healing occurs. Just as you may not consider yourself an artist, you may not think of yourself as a healer, either. You may have never used this powerful inner part of yourself consciously. But just as everyone is an artist, we know that everyone is a healer. The art we make together in the coming weeks is designed to help you get to know the healer within.

As an artist looking inward, you will be listening to what your body, mind, and spirit are telling you; expressing what you see and feel in these experiences in a caring, open, and soulful expression; and channeling the voice and hands of your healer within. You're tapping into the powerful flow of the life force, the constant act of creation that happens all the time in and around us. It's the simple, natural, and intrinsic reality of our being, which is connected to the infinite source of all life. Making art opens the flow. This method will teach you to let the natural healing process of the body and mind work as you focus on the health of your spirit.

Each time you make art, the creative self can be reborn, brand new. Each day offers new ways of being, feeling, and doing. Each day we can re-create ourselves. The process is similar to the grass that sprouts up between the cracks in the concrete. With the creative healing force, you can learn to grow new shoots and harness new forms, ideas, visions, and realities. The possibilities of expression are infinite, and this is what frees you to heal at your core.

After years of teaching people, we can confidently say that it is easier than you can imagine, but it can be a new way of making art for most people. For some, the Inner Critic can sometimes get in the way of our deepest expressions of felt-art, even for professional artists. Many people feel fear about sharing something personal with a group.

Release whatever doubts you may be holding on to. We will begin the first guided imagery, in which we journey into the past to locate the muse within and face your Inner Critic.

Before we begin this first art-healing project, there are a few things to prepare.

- Find a place to practice your art-healing.
- Find the time to practice your art-healing.
- Get some basic art supplies—your Medicine Art kit.
- Form or join an art-healing work group (optional).

## Creating an Art-Healing Space-Time in Your Life

*"Stepping into art and healing for me was like stepping into sacred space and time. I felt excited and joyful to do the process each week."*
—**Troy**, student in Spirituality and Creativity in Healthcare,
University of Florida

For many people, taking care of themselves is a crucial step in healing their pain. However, this can be hard to do sometimes—even when the decision to make yourself the focus of your healing process is so critical. This is especially true for people who care for everyone around them. Debra, a nurse, felt selfish when she made her art. She was so used to taking care of others that when she dedicated time to herself, she felt guilty. When she developed breast cancer, Debra realized that she deserved to have others take care of her; more important, she needed to finally take care of herself. For her healing process she created a piece of art with the internationally renowned sculptor Christiane Corbat. Christiane made plaster casts of the hands of each of the people taking care of her. Each person put a message of love in the plaster palms. Debra cried every time she read the messages. She realized that she deserved the wonderful care her friends, family, and caregivers were giving her. A crucial part of her art was accepting that she, the usual caregiver, needed and wanted the care.

Making art to heal is about finding an opportunity for you to do exactly what you want and need for yourself so that you can be whole. It is about you healing your life. Make yourself a priority—because you deserve it. When you care for yourself, you can give more to your family, children, friends, coworkers, community, and the environment.

One essential part of the healing process is giving yourself the time and space to create.

## *Step One: Make Time*

In an increasingly fast-paced, efficient world, time can be the most precious resource you have. Giving yourself time is the most useful healing tool. By giving yourself attention, you listen to and learn about yourself.

We recommend creating a routine around each week's material. Make these moments your own. Create art every day or every week, depending on your schedule— just make sure your time is free of distractions. In our classes, there are students who get so excited that they make art for hours, and there also are those who fit it in when they can. Don't worry if you miss days. Remember, this is for you to heal and change your life. It's not a burden, an assignment, or something you have to do. It is joy and self-discovery. It is full of life.

At first, you may need to experiment with the particular day of the week or the hour of the day. Figure out whether you prefer mornings or evenings, until you find your rhythm and pace. The simplest way is probably the best. It will grow from there. Consistency will become important once you find the best routine. This work is your gift to you. You're doing it to be healthy and feel alive, full, and creative. Value yourself enough to do it. Make this simple act as important as anything else you do in life. As we said in the introduction, you do not need to complete the process in exactly twelve weeks. If you skip weeks and then do a lot of art making, that is fine, too. As long as you complete your Medicine Art and your final project, this program will work for you.

## *Step Two: Make Sacred Space*

The next thing to do is create a physical studio that reflects your wonderful energy. It can be any kind of place or space—between the covers of your journal, the sanctuary of your bed and bedroom, a corner of the kitchen, attic, backyard shed, or garage worktable.

What is sacred space? If you were to walk on a road and find a rock, it might be an impediment that you move aside with annoyance. If you are a devout Buddhist and you learned that this was the rock that Buddha had sat on for his vision, it would be the most sacred place—a place to go to for solace or escape, full of healing energy and significance. Each person's sacred space is their own and is deeply tied to personal meaning, their own story, and what they believe in.

Sacred space is crucial in the twelve-week process. In each class we lead, all artwork is done after intentionally making sacred space. We both do different things. Michael uses prayer, incorporating sage and medicine wheels before guided imagery and art making. Mary does guided imagery, prayer, and a short art exercise with music and candles. But we never do anything in ordinary space; we work in a sacred art-healing space.

Make a space that feels different to you from your ordinary spaces. Play soft music and put candles, aromas, and objects you love in this place. Create a personal and loving boundary around yourself for privacy. It's your sacred space—your own healing temple. We guarantee that this new sacred space and time will spark memories. Images will emerge. In ordinary life you never are focused enough to be still or go inward enough to be truly creative. Intense focus and concentration create the physiology of healing and help the immune system function at its best.

### *Sacred Altars*

The process of art and healing takes place in sacred space and time. It has been done this way since ancient times and has taken many forms, from African dancing to Native American ceremonies. The process is making its way back into modern healthcare via the many Arts in Medicine programs throughout the world. We ask our students to make a sacred altar with this conscious, ancient, and wise intent. It's one of the best ways to create space in your studio, home, or hospital room—a place to "change the channel," as one student put it, and step out of the constraints of ordinary time and space.

Altars are a special kind of healing art. They hold a prayer. They can be portable. They are easily created. They make any place sacred space. In hospitals, altars also bring a sacred, religious, and spiritual component to healthcare. Making art in a sacred space brings spirituality to healing and helps illuminate the spirit.

To make your own sacred altar:

- Say a prayer to make your work powerful and healing. Choose the place in your home, office, art-healing studio, hospital room, or other spot that you love.
- Collect objects that are sacred to you, things you find meaningful, art you think is beautiful, scented candles or incense you like, and even the food you love. You can find a gift from your beloved, a photo of a child, or a photo of a departed ancestor. You can choose spiritual, religious, or iconic items that reflect your spiritual belief system: crosses, a Bible, a Buddha, Tibetan bowls, statues of gods or goddesses, bells or Native American Zuni fetishes, stones, and things from nature.
- Place them on your altar to honor your self, creativity, and spirituality.

You can also invite friends or people you work with into this sacred space. Mary's altar, for example, is next to the front door of her house, welcoming everyone who enters. It has an icon of the Blessed Mother, since she was raised Catholic. It also has a Buddha, a small Shiva and Shakti figure, Tibetan bowls and bells, and an incense holder.

When I walk by my altar it holds me for a moment, before I rush through my day. My altar is a sacred space that holds my life energetically. The altar is a place in the physical world that holds my spiritual story. I get solace from it. I add things to it; it's alive. I light my candle, say prayers, and ring the Tibetan bowl to make a sound. I light incense in morning, I look at it, and it holds meditation for me. My icons represent the many faces of God. God receives my prayers.

Before you begin your Medicine Art, make your altar and pray to bring in healing energy as you work. You can simply take one object that is most meaningful to you in your life now, say a prayer for intent, and begin. It's a simple step, but it changes everything.

## Samantha's Story: Nourishment through Painting

Samantha, a student at the Institute for Holistic Health Studies at San Francisco State University, told us about how important it was for her to make time and space for art. Long hours at work often stop art making right in its tracks, which lets the Inner Critic take root more easily, sometimes bringing depression as the person loses track of their authentic self. Samantha explained her situation:

In my junior year of college, I received a full-ride scholarship to do two years of research in mental health. I felt that earning this prestigious award was a once-in-a-lifetime opportunity, and I willingly stepped through the door, catapulting myself into the academic world. I was excited and determined to build myself as a scholar. In doing so, I became so involved with work that my creative practice, which was not valued as an important skill in my field, fell into the background. My work became my first priority, and I spent hours upon hours in a cerebral cycle of reading and writing papers, absorbing as much information as I could.

Days without my art practice turned into weeks and then months, and slowly my life became like a dry river. I was unhappy, without energy, and I felt trapped. I worked on topics that did not fuel the creative soul that I had worked so hard to enliven after past life challenges. I could not smile the same. I felt malnourished, tired, and overstressed.

I starved myself of the art I love and the practices that nourish me. I experienced a slow and gradual descent into darkness. I experienced burnout and became very ill. Illness and lack of energy forced me to slow down, step back, and listen to my body. My body, mind, and spirit told me to look in front of me. The answers to my pain had been staring at me through my research all along. I needed to make art, to paint, to come home to the practice.

I met a man who began to paint with me. Together we began a practice of painting. I painted words to remind me of who I am at my core. I painted affirmations and mantras to remind me to be myself, stay true, and be authentic.

We painted outdoors, on big walls in the city. Each time I painted, pent-up emotional experiences released from my body. The process of painting taught me to break free from these emotions and ideas that no longer served me. Painting shattered the "I'm not good enough," "You aren't worthy," "You're a failure" complexes and negativity that held me back from being who I am. Painting with him accelerated my healing by allowing me to be seen as a wounded woman healing. He was there as my healing community, honoring the work I was doing and giving support and encouragement when I found it hard to push on.

Like Samantha, we've found that when people take the time and space to focus on healing, their worlds expand. They learn to try new things and to be open to healing themselves first and foremost. They develop senses that have lain dormant, and they can see that there is a light powered by our spirits in the dark tunnel. As facilitators in the process for so many years, we find it's still a truly inspirational metamorphosis to watch. We feel very blessed to have participated in so many awakenings.

## *Art-Healing Space-Time Checklist*

Make a place in yourself, for yourself, in your schedule to make art that heals.

- Create time and space in your life.
- Make a commitment to make art to heal.
- Regard art as an important thing you do to heal yourself.
- Make yourself the focus of your healing process.
- Create a routine to make art every week.
- Create a loving boundary around yourself.
- Bless your sacred space and time with a prayer.

# Assemble Your Medicine Art Kit

As we approach our first project, you will need a few items.

## Your Art-Healing Journal

The first art-healing tool you'll need is a journal to write, sketch, and brainstorm in. We have found over the years that journaling is one of the best tools people have in covering the art-healing terrain of their lives. Your journal is essentially your mode of exploring and collecting artifacts that arise from the work you do in the coming weeks.

The journal is not just for the illustrative or literary arts. For example, if you have the temperament of a sculptor, you can muse about sculpting and sketch shapes. If you're a musician, you can write out melodies and song lyrics. Your art-healing journal is a studio unto itself, a realm to explore your thoughts, feelings, and emotions. It is a place to doodle or make collages, bounce ideas, jot down a dream or a quote you like—a home away from home. The journal is alive and will act as your muse, close friend, workshop, and exhibition site all in one.

Look around your life. Find a beautiful place where you can write each day in your journal. Find a healing environment with special objects, beautiful things, natural light, a view, and maybe music you enjoy. Find your favorite books and make them accessible to inspire you. In the beginning, being inspired by other artists or mentors who are part of your community helps. Your journal will create an energetic field where you can start to make art. Your journal is an invitation to get in touch with yourself, be in your own body, and allow your life to be the canvas of your own creativity.

Your journal will become your touchstone for the creative process. The journal is the container for your creative musings, the receptacle of the pieces of art you create, a holder, a companion and friend with a life of its own. It will also help you reflect as you write, draw, and review what you've drawn and written.

This journal will help you cultivate a simple, easy way of doing what you love and will also help you with your final project. For example, one woman decided to put pictures of her motorcycle in her journal. She drew and collected images of motorcycles. Her paintings focused on her project: making art about motorcycles. One day, she did something she'd always wanted to do: she painted her motorcycle and took a ride after the paint had dried. While writing about it in her journal, she realized she wanted to ride anywhere, anytime without plans or destinations. This changed her basic relationship with her academic and career goals. The journal helped her get in touch with the part of her that wanted to relax and simply do what she wanted each moment, without knowing where she wanted to go. Knowing who she was made this all right. Medicine Art projects are like that; you begin with an idea of what you love, and it loves you back!

We have kept journals, and so have all our students and our patients in the hospital programs. We've borne witness to so much transformation with this simple tool. Remember, the journal is not a place of judgment but one of artistic freedom. It's about opening up and letting the light within you shine through.

Mary shows you how to journal.
http://www.youtube.com/watch?v=GtvpD4Iz668&list=PLMm-0ccB
-CYpmKktLEws7WlrNyNg2QDnu&index=15

## Basic Art-Healing Supplies

This book is your perfect opportunity to go to a local art supply store and have fun. In the spirit of playfulness, pick out supplies that pop out or resonate with you—things you know you'll want to play with. Sample a variety of supplies. Look on the shelves and see what appeals to you. You may have never done this before. It may be your first time in an art store. Try not to worry, and dive in. Buy what you can afford; it doesn't need to be fancy. You don't need a lot. If you can't afford to buy supplies, be creative and inventive with recycling items you find around your home. Get some children's art materials or office supplies and use them.

When we give our classes, we bring ample amounts of the following supplies:

- A new journal of any kind
- Pens, colored pencils, crayons, pastels, erasers
- Blank scrap paper (white, colored, patterned)
- Glue, scissors, rulers, triangles, protractors
- Clay or Play-Doh
- Paint, markers, glitter, gold stars

You can also find materials you can bring new life to by reclaiming old postcards and photographs. Students of the program have collected, for example:

- Magazines and newspapers to collect pictures and words to collage for a visual diary
- Postcards, cards, or pictures from museums, art galleries, and travel
- Pictures of faces, animals, or other objects of interest
- Poems or quotes that resonate with you
- Old letters from a lover, friend, or pen pal

Make an art bin or area in your home, desk, backpack, or room. Make it easy to grab your supplies on the go.

If you're having trouble coming up with ideas for the kind of materials you'd like to use in your journal, we recommend making a list of the things you absolutely love. After you write this list, then collect photos, poems, affirmations, or quotes to adorn it.

You can also personalize your journal. Take your new art supplies and make a collage on the outside of the journal. Paint your name on the cover with acrylics, glue on letters from a magazine, and decoupage with a brush. Whatever you choose, let your journal reflect you. The whole idea is to open yourself up to being creative, to being an artist. Expand the possibilities. Experience new ways of playing music, becoming a dancer, creating a garden, buying plants to make a garden, cooking by color or smell, and using your artistry to make food. Creativity emerges when you embody your life force; your action is an expression of that experience.

Once you've collected the core components of your Medicine Art kit and start personalizing your journal, you're ready to begin the first part of this week's art-healing project.

## Week 1 Praxis

"I was afraid in the beginning that I was not an artist," said Terry, a class participant in the Shands Arts in Medicine program. He was worried about what other people thought about his artwork. Terry, at first, was like a lot of students in the program: in many people's lives, barriers and obstacles have prevented them from doing art or being creative.

Whether it was a career choice or past criticism that steered us away from a creative mind-set, almost all of us have experienced obstacles to creativity at some point. Know that these obstacles need not hold you back any longer. It's worth the risk to channel your inborn artist. You can let go of any insecurities or inhibitions. The risk of keeping an illness, depression, or lack of meaning in your life far outweighs your fear of becoming an artist. This is an opportunity to let go of your fear. What was worrisome before is not important now.

We all face the Inner Critic, that voice that tells us we're too clumsy to dance, too tone-deaf to sing, too immature to write, and so forth. The Inner Critic has an opinion about more than just your creations; it's the same voice that tells us we're not good enough or talented enough to follow our dreams. But as Terry told us, "First, I let go of my Inner Critic. As I made more and more art, I was not concerned about what anyone thought of my art. The honest, judgment-free spirit gave me courage."

Now is the time in your life to tell the Inner Critic to take a rest and let you be who you are. This is a crucial general and basic step to creativity in the art and healing process—a judgment-free, loving, and supportive process. You do it to heal yourself, others, or the earth, and this is what makes it truly beautiful.

## Guided Imagery: Meeting Your Inner Artist and Releasing Your Inner Critic

As mentioned, from our experience, healing art is most powerful when it is made in sacred space. When we do this process with our classes, we begin each week with a meditation to ask for help from religious figures or energies. Then we make a protective, safe, and loving space to make Medicine Art. We will do this before beginning every week's praxis.

Go to the quiet space you've designated as your art-healing space. Relax and let your breathing slow down. Take the time to sit in silence for a moment. Ask a higher consciousness to come to you. It can be a religious figure you believe in, a Higher Power, nature, an ancestor, a guide, or anything that helps you see deeper into your life. Ask it to bless you in your art and healing work. Give thanks and gratitude. Ask the higher consciousness to guide your hands and to send you images to make art that will heal you, others, your community, or the earth. Then you are ready to begin to make art to heal.

## The Inner Artist

Close your eyes, rest, and relax. Let the tension in your life escape as you take slow, deep breaths. Feel your abdomen rise several inches as you breathe in, and feel it fall several inches as you breathe out. With each breath, let yourself get larger and larger in your mind's eye, expanding beyond your body. As you expand, imagine the spaces between your cells also getting larger as you inhale. Allow the spaces between your cells to fill with light and energy as you breathe in. The light can be white, blue, green—any color you see fit.

Now that you are saturated with light, relax even more. Let your breathing get deeper. Your abdomen rises and falls as you breathe, taking you deeper. Let your mind take you back to a point in your childhood or in your life, a moment of making art that was full of happiness and joy, when you felt the free of constraint and fully expressive artistically in your life—whether it was when dancing, playing music, drawing, painting, writing poetry, or play-acting. Go back to the time when you actually lived making art, a time when you allowed yourself to be truly creative and satisfied.

Go back to that artful moment and enter your body. Recall how it felt. Remember the world around you; be in the situation where you were making art, the way you experienced it. Look at your hands and feel the materials you held, remember your thoughts, and experience how excited you felt. Be with this memory in totality. Rest in its innocence and beauty. Feel how wonderful it was. See the art you loved to make. Meet your Inner Artist, a spirit you may have not encountered for a while.

## The Inner Critic

Was there a dream you had before life became so formed? What did you desire when you were uninhibited and still thought anything was possible? Was there a moment when you were told you could not do something? Perhaps someone told you that you could not draw a straight line or that you needed to stay between the lines as you colored. Perhaps someone told you that you were too ugly or clumsy to dance, that you could not sing on key or play the piano, or that you were lazy and did not practice enough. Maybe this person was a parent, teacher, or another student whose criticism made you shut down as you drew, danced, sang, or spoke from your heart. Maybe the critic was not another person but yourself; you may have felt embarrassed in class, comparing yourself with others.

Picture other moments in your life when you did something beautiful and were told it was not the right thing to do. Did someone say that your music would never make you money? Maybe they said that you should not be an artist but a lawyer, banker, or doctor instead. In your mind's eye, picture the person who told you these things. Hear and see them criticize you. How did you feel in your body? See, smell, and sense the scene clearly.

If you went to art school or took art classes, you can also picture moments in a critique. You made something you believed in and loved and were told it was "not art," would not sell, or was not what people were doing now.

Whatever your past, go into that moment and picture it unfolding. See the person who told you that you can't make art. Remember what they said, what happened, and how you felt in that moment. Search your senses and memory until it's real. This voice you hear is the voice of the Inner Critic, which keeps you from being free, creative, and authentically *you*, without the constraints of society.

Now we will release the Inner Critic. Let it go. Imagine that you can put the Inner Critic in a room, a box, or a soundproof closet or on another planet—anywhere but where you're making art. Keep them quiet and away from you as you make art to heal. Thank them for the help they give you in keeping you safe, if you wish, but tell them you are making art to heal and you don't need that voice now. You are doing exactly what you need to do—confronting your fears and exposing your suffering. The Inner Critic can leave and let you be. Watch them leave, watch them go far away or into the box or room until they disappear.

Pause for a moment. Let this image go. Relax and take a long, deep breath.

Now come back to where you are. Feel your body and its denseness. Feel the chair, floor, or bed. Bring with you your feelings and impressions of the guided imagery. We'll be doing much more guided imagery to widen this space in the coming weeks.

### *Medicine Art: Draw from Your Guided Imagery about Your Inner Artist and Critic*

For your first Medicine Art project, think of the guided imagery of meeting your Inner Artist and releasing the Inner Critic. Draw, watercolor, or paint what you saw. You can draw the figure, words, or paint an image that came to you in your vision; you can portray one scene or make sequential art. You can also collage, draw stick figures, or mold a clay figure.

You can also draw or make a container for your Critic. You can make something elaborate or put them on a page in your journal where they can't get out. Put walls around them. You can draw a prison or even put them in a rocket ship. Send them away for the time you are making art to heal.

One idea comes from a woman in Michael's class who used her Critic's container as her final Medicine Art project. Over the weeks, she constructed a beautiful, elaborate box within a box, complete with matching locks and keys. In the smaller box, she put pictures of her Inner Critic along with the words the Critic had said. For her presentation, she locked the boxes in front of the class. Everyone cheered. It was as if she had put everyone's Inner Critic away.

You can also focus on your Inner Artist by creating art that explores what media you like and what you might want to use in your final Medicine Art project.

If nothing specific comes to you from the guided imagery right away, just doodle. Do whatever art comes to you in the moment. You can begin by starting to draw colors, abstract shapes, and color washes. Remember, there is no right or wrong art. You do not need to show your work to anyone if you don't want to. The intention for this first piece of Medicine Art is to begin embracing and trusting your Inner Artist while letting go of the Inner Critic.

Feel free to take pauses and then come back. Work at your own pace. If you want to, share your creation with your art-healing group. If you are working by yourself, write about the experience in your journal. The important thing is to trust what came to you during guided imagery—without judgment.

### Making Art from Guided Imagery

- Experiment with different materials: watercolors, collage, paints, colored pencils, and/or crayons.
- Remember an image you were attracted to in the guided imagery and start drawing it.
- Spend a half hour drawing what you were attracted to.
- Play music to help you relax.
- If you did not see something you'd like to draw, draw anything you want to. Start with color and then create a shape. Let it grow.
- There is no right or wrong thing to draw.
- This is not a test or a project for anyone to see; it is art to heal.
- Don't judge. Just draw.

## Summary of Week 1

- Create an art-healing sacred time-space.
- Assemble your Medicine Art kit.
- Meet your Inner Artist.
- Let go of your Inner Critic.
- Draw from your guided imagery and journal about it.
- Complete your first Medicine Art project based on the guided imagery and journal entry.

# WEEK 2

# MERGING YOUR INNER ARTIST AND HEALER

*The artist and healer are one, just as the rhythm of a heartbeat is one with
the rhythm of the earth. Breathe in the universal flow as it opens us
to the fullness of who we really are as artist-healers.*

Welcome to the second week of using Art as a Healing Force, in which we awaken your Inner Healer with the exquisite beauty of art that resonates in body, mind, and spirit for life-changing effects.

Learning to make art to heal is different from learning to become a professional artist. It is an invitation to use whatever kind of art you want to open yourself to the vitality within you. Keep in mind that healing can be different from curing; sometimes healing takes place during a life-threatening illness, although the disease is not cured.

Over the years, we've found that when profound personal art reaches into the core of a person's soul—the singing of a song, writing of a poem, or painting of a picture—it can be as medicinal as a regimen of pills or a session with a therapist. People in Arts in Medicine programs throughout the country have discovered this powerful way to heal that changes their lives.

Even those who carry wounds they think will never heal can develop tools for healing the deepest of scars—warriors returning from the combat zone, people with cancer, or a community trying to heal itself after a shared tragedy. Take Laura, for example. She was a student of Michael's in his Art as a Healing Force university class in Bolinas.

Laura did not speak much during class and didn't reveal much personally. But on the last day she changed us all.

## Laura's Story: Dancing in the Darkness

When it was Laura's turn to present her final project, she stood up in the circle, paused, and looked at everyone. She reached into a bag and draped colored scarves around her body while moving to the center of the circle. She told the class that she was going to do a dance to heal a violent rape.

You could see the reactions and hear faint gasps from the class as they comprehended what would be happening. They understood that they would be witness to a powerful event.

Then Laura started to dance. As she moved, we were taken by her power and beauty in this sacred moment. The first small movement was like a wind blowing through our space. Her arm moved, and we all moved with it. She carried her holiness like a priestess of ancient times.

She moved faster. Her energy rose, the colors blended, and she seemed to take power from the sky and from the earth, as if ancient spirits were helping her heal deeply.

As she danced, she rose in power. Then her motions became violent. It was as if she were pushing away the energy of the rape. We could all feel how the healing and energy came up as she danced. She healed all the women in the room—and the men, too—with her powerful, uplifting dance. We were speechless. Quiet Laura had spoken volumes. She wrote to Michael about what the healing had meant and how it played into her recovery:

I was struggling. Struggling in my relationship, struggling to move past events that had happened to me years prior to the Art as a Healing Force class, and struggling to step into my power as a woman who had survived rape. I couldn't see myself as a survivor, only as a victim. I was a victim to the men that had done such an atrocious thing to a young girl. I was a victim of a family that turned a blind eye because they didn't—couldn't—know how to react. I was crumbling inside, but I easily put on the façade that I was fine. I did that for thirteen years.

I had spent many of those years covering up the pain with alcohol, drugs, and sex. As I grew out of that and met my partner, I was open with him about my experience. He was so supportive. As years went on, I felt residual pain. I didn't know how to allow myself to properly heal. I began to seek guidance from shamans, talk therapy, and journaling. It never seemed to go anywhere. I continued to find myself in a place of shame, self-judgment, and insecurity. It began to drastically affect my relationship. We decided to part ways for a while, to my despair.

I decided the following fall that I would enroll in the Art as a Healing Force class. It sounded good. The art of dance had always been a way for me to lose myself in song and movement and feel my body in a different way. I had never danced with the intention of translating my internal struggle.

Little did I know that this class would gently pull me out of my darkness and ask me to dance with the memories. I finally allowed myself to begin the process of truly letting go.

Rape and sexual abuse are the subject of many final projects, even though they can be the hardest stories to tell. The "darkness," as Laura calls it, can be a deep source of hurt within that people often bury under the fast-paced rigor of our increasingly complex daily lives—that is, until it starts manifesting itself mentally and physically. In spite of this, art can be a powerful channel for healing deep scars.

We'll be talking more about Laura and her story in the weeks ahead. We'll look more deeply at the issue of facing our own version of "darkness." For now, Laura's dance shows what art-healing is really all about: letting the soulful, courageous, artist-healer emerge in your life.

## Art and Healing as Lovers

Rachel Naomi Remen, clinical professor of Family and Community Medicine at UCSF School of Medicine, wrote, "At the deepest level, the creative process and the healing process arise from a single source," but we often forget that the first artist and the first healer were one and the same. Healing with art originated in the warm embrace of a sacred union—the vision that Michael had witnessed on Mount Tamalpais.

From the dawn of human consciousness, making art and healing were considered one act in many cultures—inseparable, unified, and completely in one ceremony. The first art-healing practices were music and dance ceremonies in hunter-gatherer cultures.

These first peoples believed that a healing spirit was freed from within a person by participating in profound, rhythmic music and artful expression. Many cultures around the world believe spirits cause illness and dancing takes them away.

The Kalahari Bushmen call this "boiling energy." The Bushmen are a people who thrived in the African desert as hunter-gatherers until the 1950s, when they adopted agriculture. Anthropologists believe that looking at the way our ancestors lived may yield clues about how ancient peoples used art and healing for millions of years—before the knowledge is lost.

Richard Katz of the Harvard University Kalahari Research Group visited the Bushman people and wrote about their healing dance rituals in his book *Boiling Energy*. He described how the whole community would participate in all-night dances that lasted several nights a week. They believed that dance freed up the boiling energy within them and was the way to heal. During the dance ritual their bodies became incredibly hot, and enormous energy came up from within them. These techniques often caused their illness to subside. Sometimes they would go into a trance after dancing for hours, and people around them would touch them and help them.

This community healing ritual was an ordinary part of the Bushmen's lives and was not something special or artificial. Medicine Art was part of their worldview. Today human culture has changed, since everyone in the community is an artist-healer. Now naturally gifted healers such as medicine women and men called shamans work for the group.

Traditional shamans sang, danced, made music, and drummed; made costumes, rattles, and headdresses; and led the audience or participants in rituals. The shaman is a specialist in those ritual practices of hunter-gatherer communities. However, art and healing were still one concept. The art was still transformational. Art was made to heal, bless the hunt, heal the community, and change the world.

Eventually in tribal cultures across the globe, the sacred rituals and shamans soon faded away. There are still individuals among us who dance, make amulets, sing, go into trances, and see spirits in the inner world. They are the remaining shamans, priestesses, and medicine people. The separation of art and healing has progressed. Now we have medications and surgery, and art is seen as a special talent for a minority of people and shown at galleries or museums.

We believe it is time for art and healing to unite again. Everyone can take back the role of shaman or artist-healer. The transformational process is too powerful to keep in the realm of the specialist. Our bodies, homes, communities, and earth need everyone to become artist-healers.

We can draw from the myraid art-healing traditions of cultures all over the world. Christian and Buddhist art also works on the principle that meditating on images or listening to certain sounds puts a person in a sacred healing state. There are cathedrals, sacred music, iconography of Jesus and Mary, and Tibetan thangka paintings of the healing Tara. In Lourdes, France, and Tinos, Greece, the Virgin Mary heals. Paintings in the Church are meditation objects for people to enhance healing.

Just as Laura was able to tap into her own kind of boiling energy, we want you to concentrate on the boiling energy within you. Start focusing on it through this week's art project. Looking at the healing dances of ancient cultures, there are several important lessons that still apply today.

- *Participation is key.* The dance (art) was done by everyone. No singular central figure did something to the sick person. There were people who led the dance, but the healing was accomplished by the dancing itself. Physical movements freed the healing energy. The dancers essentially became their own healing artists by making art that freed their inner healer, and they shared this with the whole group. Boiling energy bubbled up from each of them. When you make art and concentrate deeply, your creative trance can take you to a place inside you that's full of ideas, visions, or thoughts. These are the meditations you can sample from to create a work of healing art to share with others in the world.

- *Art-healing is a single concept.* In the process, people did not separate art and healing. Their healing dancing was simply a "freeing" of energy, a transformation. It was not for entertainment, although it certainly was exciting. Dance and healing were one. We cannot say the dance *caused* healing; it simply was healing. This sharing was seen as sacred, too, as part of the spiritual life of the community.

As mentioned, there are myriad traditions of using images of sacred figures to heal. Feel free to incorporate them into your own healing work and to share your inspiration with your art-healing group. Regardless of your beliefs or background, when you make your own art to heal, you bring the energy of the healing image to life, just as the artist-healers of old once did.

# The Physiology of Art as a Healing Force

Art heals. This statement is not only substantiated by time-tested traditions but it's also a scientifically verified fact. There are thousands of research studies about how creativity, art, and spiritual experiences help heal physical and mental illnesses and promote personal growth. Because art and healing change the body's physiology, it is effective in physical healing. A comprehensive research report in the *Journal of Public Health* looked at all the recent research and described proven ways that art heals. The results showed that art helped many parameters that promote healing and quality of life.

In many research studies, art and healing has been shown to:

- Enhance social support, psychological strength, and help people gain new insights into their illness experience
- Help people express complex emotions (anxiety, isolation, fear)
- Help people cope with trauma
- Help people experience joy
- Help people connect with the spirit
- Ease depression
- Enhance spirituality
- Reduce stress, depression, and anger
- Increase immune function and endorphins
- Alter perception of pain and decrease the need for pain medication
- Induce mind-body changes that speed and promote healing

The science doesn't lie: when you make art with the intent to heal either yourself or someone else—giving up your Inner Critic and inviting your Inner Artist to merge with your Inner Healer—you immediately shift from a physiology of fear, anxiety, competition, judgment, and stress to a physiology of love, caring, and healing.

How does this psychological-turned-physiological process work? This shift that can occur in your body via a shift in your state of mind is the product of your autonomic nervous system (ANS), the part of the nervous system that controls functions in the body like heart rate, digestion, breathing, salivation, perspiration, pupil dilation, and sexual arousal. The ANS has a yin-yang design, with two opposing branches: the sympathetic system and the parasympathetic system.

- Sympathetic arousal speeds up the heart rate, increases breathing, sends blood to the large muscles, and floods the body with adrenaline and stress hormones, thus creating a physiology of alertness. Facing down a snarling dog would set your sympathetic system on full alert.

- The stimulation of the parasympathetic branch of the ANS, on the other hand, results in relaxation, tissue rebuilding, immune system enhancement, and healing. When you're out of danger, the feeling of safety relieves tension in your body and puts you back in a natural, healing state of release.

This cycle is called the arousal/release cycle. It charts each person's way of reacting to any exciting event.

Most autonomous functions were thought to be involuntary, but we now know that many ANS actions are affected by the mind and consciousness. Images you experience are associated with the firing of neurons in the right brain; this activates the hypothalamus, which controls your ANS. When you do guided imagery that leads to an art-healing project, you're consciously activating the types of images that are homeostatic, or self-healing, to flow through your brain and body. It's a way of re-patterning old neural structures in a healing, reaffirming way and creating new synapses.

You already have an innate knowledge of how this process works. An image in your mind can dramatically affect your body, changing your physiology and blood flow to specific areas of your body within seconds. Sexual fantasy is a classic example. When you picture your lover or imagine making love, your body becomes aroused. Your conscious mind knows that it's just a fantasy, but images from your right brain make your body think it's merging with your lover. For your sexual self, this imaginary image starts in your brain but moves to your entire physical being. Your breathing speeds up, heart rate rises, eyes dilate, and sexual organs fill with blood and fluids. Your emotions change. You feel excitement, dreaminess, and tingling. Pulsations ripple through your body in waves of nerve- and hormone-induced arousal. We take this process for granted, although it is very complicated and beautiful. By imagining a loving or sexual image, you can feel the blood flow changing your body chemistry. Whole cascades of physiological changes are initiated by a mental image or memory.

Of course, the imagery doesn't have to be sexual. In fact, the image you hold in your brain does not have to be an object that exists in the outer world for it to have an effect on your body. All that's important is that you see it with your mind's eye and imagine it clearly. The memory of something embarrassing happening to you in public, for example, can make you blush, even if it happened years ago. Your heart rate accelerates, breathing speeds up, blood flow to your digestive organs slows, and blood flow to your big muscles increases.

The more you can balance the arousal and release, the more mastery you have over this system. Medicine Art is an easy and accessible way of exercising this ability. The same principle holds true for a profound scene or image from your life that can either make you laugh or cry. That memory creates a physiological response so strong that your experience of the imagery is not only a mental process but a bodily experience as well.

Seeing yourself going places, doing things, uncovering truths, and helping others is an important part of the art-healing process. It's why we have our students envision spiritual experiences as often as they can. When you picture a scene that is beautiful and moving, your body reacts with joy and relaxation. You don't have to be there; your body will react naturally, as if it's there, and go into healing physiology.

The physiology of deep relaxation and healing that results from this state is similar to the physiology of prayer and meditation. This has been known since Dr. Herbert Benson at the Behavioral Medicine Clinic at Harvard University Medical School wrote about it in his classic book *The Relaxation Response*. He showed that meditation alone lowers blood pressure, heart rate, and breathing rate, and can be used as a primary therapy for heart disease patients. Today Dr. Dean Ornish uses meditation and yoga as a major part of his heart disease regimen to reduce stress. He also uses it for its spiritual focus to reduce alienation and promote feelings of connectedness and oneness. Making art to heal is even more powerful because it involves all the senses at once, helps change brainwave states, and deals with both the outer world and inner world. That is why so many cultures have used art and healing as ceremony to heal and why it's such a crucial tool on our twelve-week course.

When a person translates healing images in the mind to making art—painting, dancing, journaling, playing music, sculpting a pot for your lover to put flowers in, building an herb garden for your elderly neighbor, or dancing with your children while they fight an illness—these types of art-healing activities produce a deep level of healing concentration and mindful muscle movements. If the image is one of joy or a release of tension, the body is put in a healing state through the hypothalamic pathways of the parasympathetic nervous system. The heart rate and breathing slow, blood pressure drops, blood goes to the intestines, and the whole physiology changes. This process takes the person's whole attention, freeing them from their worries and concerns of the external world. It happens automatically. The artist-healer does not need to do anything except focus intensely. The ancient neural pathways of the mind take over; you're taken "elsewhere" to a mental state of pure concentration that resembles meditation.

This simplified model of the anatomy of the art-healing system gives us an idea of how the mind is connected to the body and how images and muscle movements can stimulate our entire being. By way of the relaxation response, the images become automatically self-healing. This process can involve any of the five senses or all of them at once:

- Visual
- Auditory
- Sensory
- Olfactory
- Gustatory

The images involve the firing of neurons in different areas of the brain. The firing neurons, the nets of cascading activity, connect to the body in three simple ways: (1) they change nerve impulses to the organs, (2) they change hormonal balance, and (3) they change neurotransmitters in the brain.

When these visions come to the surface of our consciousness from the inner self and are released, it can be deeply healing. For example, when a person sees the Blessed Mother, they hold the image of her in their brain and feel it in their body.

Mary, for example, recalls entering the Chartres Cathedral and seeing the Black Madonna. The experience of imagery and light was so powerful that she felt her whole body "shift." She recognized that the experience was ancient, resonating within every pilgrim who had ever visited the Blessed Mother. She still feels that resonance today when she conjures the image of the Virgin in that massive cathedral.

## Our Built-In Pharmacy

### Neurochemicals

Images in your mind's eye cause specific areas of the brain to release endorphins and other neurotransmitters. This release affects brain cells and the cells of your immune system by relieving pain and making the immune system function more efficiently. Killer T-cells eat cancer cells; white blood cells attack viruses; and the body's ability to respond to illness changes.

When a person has a profound, passionate experience while dancing, making music, or experiencing an image that is freeing and joyful, the body actually changes its physiology to heal itself. The release of the endorphins when we experience a vision of spirit is deeply pleasurable. It is like the way a person feels when they are exercising. The endorphins are like opiates or other mind-altering drugs. They make a person feel expanded, connected, at one, relaxed, vibrating, tingling, and peaceful.

In a real sense, the release of endorphins during prayer and spiritual visions may be *the* major healing force. It is psychoneuroimmunology at its best. Psychoneuroimmunology is a term that puts together *psycho* for the mind, *neuro* for the nerve nets of the brain, and *immuno* for the immune system. It describes how thoughts or images in the mind affect our health.

## *Hormones*

As the imagery of threat or the spiritual vision lights up the neural nets in the brain, a hormonal flood bathes every cell in our bodies via the hypothalamus, sending messages to the adrenal glands to release epinephrine, adrenaline, and other hormones, which travel throughout the body and are picked up by receptors. This process causes some cells to contract and others to relax; some act, while others rest.

Our entire physiology is changed a second time by an image or movement held in our consciousness. The second change is chemical, resulting from hormonal shifts. It is slower but just as profound. It affects almost every cell in the body. Oxytocin, for example, the "love hormone," is released when you imagine a loving field around you. This hormone promotes feelings of love, peace, connectedness, and healing and adds to the physiological effect of guided imagery of the heart and gratitude.

### Artist-Healer Profile: Institute of HeartMath— The Intelligence of the Heart

When the ANS produces the physiology of "fight or flight" or of deep healing, the heart is intimately involved. The heart rate speeds up with stress and slows with healing, but science now knows there is much more to it than this. New science of the heart is being pioneered at the exciting Institute of HeartMath in California, where researchers are developing a deeper understanding of heart intelligence and the importance of the heart in healing.

Heart intelligence is both a new phenomenon and an ancient one. People speak of the wisdom of the heart: follow your heart, listen to your heart. Now modern scientific research is finding out that the heart sends more information to the body than the brain does. In a way, the heart itself is like a brain.

The Institute of HeartMath conducts research on heart coherence, which uses the relaxation response via the parasympathetic nervous system to decrease stress. Heart coherence is basically about mastering the variable rate between your heartbeats. When people are stressed, their heart rate is chaotic and variable. This fast and slow rhythm can be transformed with meditation, breathing, and heart focus to coherence. Using awareness of the heart rhythm produces a healthy heartbeat. Then the rate between heartbeats becomes constant. Heart coherence puts people in the physiological state that decreases stress and their reaction to stress for powerful healing.

Robert Browning, director of HeartMath, and his staff teach people and healthcare programs around the country about the basic techniques of counteracting stress with heart focusing exercises that return the heart to coherence. They work with doctors, nurses, military personnel, and others.

HeartMath also has devices that measure the electromagnetic field of the heart and has found that the field radiates three to five feet outside the body, like the signal from a human radio tower. Looking at our body in this way, we see how creativity is based on a heart-centered expanded view. The human is conscious light energy—consciousness—and has a mind, body, and spirit. Many healing artists, such as painter Alex Grey, consider the human as wholeness, unity, and harmony of body, mind, and spirit. No matter what, you are whole as a spiritual being. Every human generates an electromagnetic field of heart energy that can be filled with light, love, and spirit.

We will use this electromagnetic heart energy force as part of your journey to heal. In our twelve-week process, we'll use some basic tools from HeartMath and heart research. Quick heart coherence practices include living from your heart center, breathing into your heart, and invoking gratitude and appreciation. This optimizes a physiological shift, so the heart settles and the rhythm becomes peaceful and regular. The heart then syncs with the rhythm of life and the universal heartbeat that pulses within each human, each animal, and even the earth itself. The heart has a deep intelligence in this way, one that is similar in strength to the human brain. Its characteristics can be enhanced by making deeply healing art.

# Week 2 Praxis

The images of scenes you hold in your mind turn into healing art, change nerve impulses in the body, and bring hormonal balance to each cell in your body. Simply put, a healing image manifested in reality for the good of yourself or another results in a ripple effect of healing physiology in our bodies.

For this guided imagery exercise, make yourself comfortable. You can be sitting or lying down. You'll want to loosen tight clothing and leave your legs and arms uncrossed. Close your eyes and open yourself to the experience as we re-marry art and healing.

## *Guided Imagery: Uniting Your Inner Artist and Healer*

Let your breathing slow down. Take several deep breaths. Let your abdomen rise as you breathe in and fall as you let your deep breath out. As you breathe in and out, you will become more and more relaxed.

You may feel sensations of tingling or buzzing; you may feel heaviness or lightness; or you may feel your boundaries loosening and your edges softening. If you do, let those feelings increase.

Let your feet and legs relax. Feelings of relaxation spread upward to your thighs and pelvis. Open your pelvis, relax your abdomen, and let your belly expand. Release your stress, pain, or suffering with every breath you take. Now allow your chest to relax, your heart rate and breathing slow down. Let your arms relax and then your hands. Relax your neck, head, face, and eyelids.

With your mind's eye, see a horizon. Everything is blackness. Let these feelings of relaxation spread throughout your body. If you wish, you can count your breaths and let your relaxation deepen with each breath. Feel your body. It is tingling, full of energy. This is the healing, your boiling energy.

Now see yourself making the kind of art you love most. You may envision yourself painting, dancing, writing poems, or playing music. Whatever it is, see yourself as an artist. See your Inner Artist making art. You may remember moments of making art, when you took photographs, danced, or played music. Take those beautiful memories and let them grow. See the memories and then see something far greater. See yourself creating art in the present moment. Imagine yourself making beautiful, emotional, spiritual art. Feel yourself as the incredible artist you are. You may see colorful energy around you.

Now, in your mind's eye, find your Inner Healer. See the part of your body that heals yourself, has an immune system, and makes new cells after an injury. Look inside and observe your immune system, hormones, beating heart, and breathing. You have the ability to heal from injury, illness, and trauma. Remember all the times you have healed and feel the power you have to heal yourself. Imagine healing yourself, others, and the earth. Envision your hands, your energy field. See yourself bringing the creative energy of the earth, the sky, God, and a higher consciousness into your body; then let it out. Embrace the beauty and power of your Inner Healer. Feel its energy and vibration level. You may experience the presence of ancestors, guides, angels, or spiritual figures who give you energy.

Now let your Inner Artist and Inner Healer come together. They are one. Allow the Artist to slide over the Healer. Let them merge and pop together as one. Whatever you see and feel is fine. Just let the Inner Artist and Inner Healer become one.

If you don't see anything, that is fine too. The transformation is happening inside, beyond words and visions. Trust the process, and it will be. Now see what presences are around you. They will help you be the newly combined Artist-Healer. You may see your ancestors, a grandparent, religious figures, your guides, spirit animals, your teachers, or people who love you. See what presences are with you in your spiritual journey. A higher consciousness helps heal with love and illuminate your spirit.

Realize that your work is sacred. It is a gift to your community and to the earth. As you surrender, let yourself be loose. Relax deeper. Do not be afraid. You are in the hands of guides, ancestors, and sacred teachers. You are weightless, falling into deepest space. Surrender to something much greater and older than your body.

When you are ready, come back from the vision to your surroundings. Return to the place where you are doing the exercise. First move your feet and then your hands. Mindfully experience the feeling of the movement. Press your feet down onto the floor, grounding yourself. Feel the pressure on the bottom of your feet and the solidity of the earth. Feel your backside on the chair or the floor; feel your weight pressing downward. Bring all of your self back into your physical body. Come back into your body, solidly and completely. Open your eyes. Look around you. Stand up and stretch. Move your body and feel it move.

Now come back, an Artist-Healer, ready to carry the experience of this exercise into your life. Each time you repeat this guided imagery exercise, we guarantee you'll feel stronger and be able to see deeper into yourself.

Mary shares a centering exercise and singing bowl meditation to bring in the light of art and healing.
http://www.youtube.com/watch?v=tHV2p5a7y6E&list=PLMm-0ccB -CYpmKktLEws7WlrNyNg2QDnu&index=14

### *Medicine Art: Draw from Your Guided Imagery about Your Inner Artist and Healer*

Take out your journal and art supplies and write, draw, paint, or collage what you saw during your guided imagery about your Inner Artist and Inner Healer becoming one. This is also your chance to see more deeply who your own inner Artist-Healer is. Is it a dancer or a painter? What does that new figure look like? A warrior for peace? A moon goddess? A shamanic healer? Do you see yourself healing yourself, others, community? There are no limits when life becomes your art. Have fun and find out what you look like in your sacred inner space.

Brittany, a student in Mary's class in Spirituality and Healthcare at the University of Florida, describes and talks about her body-tracing Medicine Art.
http://www.youtube.com/watch?v=Eqh5OHkmu0c&list=PLMm-0ccB -CYpmKktLEws7WlrNyNg2QDnu&index=13

## Summary of Week 2

The transformational effect of the art-healing process happens in three steps:

1. The person has the healing vision as a thought, image, or movement initiated by the creative process.
2. A message is sent to the cells by a nerve impulse, a hormone, or a neurotransmitter.
3. This shift in physiology bolsters your body's immune system. The cells become activated. They may react by eating a cancer cell or virus, sending blood to an area of illness, or relaxing and tensing.

This week:

- Do the guided imagery for making your Inner Artist and Inner Healer one.
- Draw from your guided imagery, letting your physiology be changed by the images that come to you. Use your art as an outlet for these feelings.

# WEEK 3

# THE SPIRIT IN ART HEALING

*The journey of this lifetime can be transformed as we create
sacred spiritual space and call a Higher Power to watch over us—
for we are never alone.*

Welcome to our third week of using Art as a Healing Force. We hope you had a powerful second week and are excited to expand your healing art practice. This week you will tell the story of your own spiritual history. We include this in the twelve-week program to honor our own spiritual journey and to create a collective to honor all spiritual traditions.

It is no accident we have come together to use art and healing to incorporate your spirituality and creativity. Our intention is to integrate your spiritual journey into your life so that it's a major thread that permeates your whole life. Art and healing illuminate the spirit. Research has shown that art heals by promoting spiritual experience. The story of your spiritual journey will help make your own light brighter.

Your spiritual journey is your life work. If you are a nurse, an artist, a counselor, a gardener, an engineer, a doctor, part of your spiritual destiny is this work. This chapter is about opening up your spirituality to interface with your whole life. For example, when you decided on your work, that was your calling. It was what your spirit longed to do.

This week we will also give you some exciting tools to expand your way of using art to achieve spiritual transcendence.

## The Infinite Field of Energy We Live In

As a dancer-in-residence, Inna Dagman described the place spirit had in the art-healing process: "A person might say that they are not creative, but as the weeks go by, something shifts, and all this beautiful creativity begins to flow from a place that was previously unacknowledged. That sacred spring opens up every time there is an invitation to create with the intent to heal, to hear the voice of one's spirit."

Art-healing is about recognizing the energetic body in addition to the physical one. Many artists have explored this energetic realm, from Hildegard von Bingen's illustration that represented human beings in an infinite field of unified consciousness, to the *Sacred Mirrors* paintings by visionary artist Alex Grey that show the chakras and lattices of universal consciousness.

As energetic beings and bodies of light, we reside in an infinite field of energy. This is really the "body" we work when we make healing art. We tap into the experience of being with our energetic creative selves. We are not in stagnant time but fluid. We tap into a source of higher consciousness within ourselves.

In our programs, we make art for healing with consciousness and intentionality. We make healing art with a divine presence that creates, sustains, and organizes the universe. We tap into our own awareness and connection to this higher divine reality. We do this through centering exercises, breathing exercises, heart centering, and guided imagery. Within these moments, you can let go of inner chatter and acknowledge yourself in gratitude. The most important thing in this process is to give yourself the time to pay attention, love yourself, and honor who you are as a human being. That's what creativity does. That is why intention is important; the experience of yourself is the experience.

When you make art to heal, you are more than your body, more than material, machinery, or physical form. You move into an understanding of your humanness. Consciousness is part of your work. Emotions, meanings, attitudes, and perceptions are part of your work. This new view, an emerging physiology of body, mind, and spirit in tune with one another, is manifested by creativity. We move into a transcendental place of consciousness where we are beings of light and we are all one. You dissolve into a pure light body where you are part of a lattice of love. This is a nonlocal consciousness, the source of a healing force.

Creativity is a transpersonal energetic experience. You, as the healing artist, are part of an experience based on the worldview that everything is connected. You invite all ways of knowing—spiritual, technical, emotional, and physical.

This kind of creativity is dynamic and open to every human. It provides an opportunity for manifesting change. It always heals. Healing may occur without curing, but it always touches your core. Creativity is an act of reverence and happens within the sacred space of your own being. It is life-giving and life-enriching. Our creativity is a call to deeper consciousness and an intentional, authentic choice to heal ourselves.

## The Spirit of Art

Creativity is the expression of the universal creative force, and universal love is its source. Many people see this infinite source of love as a higher consciousness. The higher consciousness can be defined as whatever you see as the infinite, unexplainable, and incomprehensible nature of a higher being or a greater force. As the higher consciousness flows into us, we express the infinite creative energy of that love as art. Art, in a way, is the higher consciousness of love speaking through us. This is the nature of the mystery of life.

We can question this mystery by asking, Who are we? What is life? How do we belong? Creativity reveals the essence of our belonging. Creativity expresses the uniqueness of the infinite field that resides within you. Essentially, a creative pulse within each person is the manifestation of the force of the infinite field. This expression is sacred.

Art leads us to the emergence of the sacred process: life itself. Using art as a healing force is about living and expressing the innate energy within. Creativity taps into the natural, powerful flow of this energy. When we make art, we invite the higher consciousness of love to flow into our personal process and be born, known, and shared. Everyone is an artist. Everyone is creative. We create ourselves each day, each moment. The higher consciousness flows through us.

The most potent healing methodology today combines creativity and spirituality to heal the soul. Health futurists, like Leland Kaiser at University of Colorado at Denver, tell us that the most powerful healing works at the level of spirit to heal the body. This work is taking place in major medical centers in spirituality and healthcare groups nationwide. There are now more than seventy-five programs of this kind in major medical schools. More than half of all hospitals have art and healing programs as well; this is transforming healing as we know it. Our Art as a Healing Force program is your doorway into this exciting world.

How can you use your own creative and spiritual life to heal? How can you tap into the wisdom of your own soul? How can two simple interventions—creativity and guided imagery—dramatically affect your health? Arts in Medicine has the answers to those questions. New studies have shown that a person who had surgery or was in critical care checked out of the hospital one day earlier and needed less narcotic pain medication if they viewed a painting of a landscape on the wall across from their bed or did a fifteen-minute guided imagery with a CD or audio download. This is an astonishing example of the enormous power of creativity and spirituality in healing. Patients with cancer who used art had a better quality of life with less pain, fewer side effects from treatment, and a better attitude toward healing.

Leland Kaiser says we are at a breaking point in medicine, a critical time in which a whole mind-set about how people look at medicine is changing. This pivotal moment is occurring as a crucial convergence of medicine, art, and spirituality. Coming together, these fields will transform how medicine is practiced and how people heal. Health theorists often call this "the plus 100 effect." By that they mean that if a patient uses mind and spirit to heal, healing is 100 percent more effective than if they don't. Health futurists believe it is an important part of the future of healthcare delivery in the twenty-first century.

This convergence is a mark of maturity in medicine, art, and spirituality. The fields have grown and become independent; they now need to unify to expand. Creativity and spirituality provide us with a new model for health that is multidimensional and much broader than the present model based on the body alone. Creativity and spirituality are emerging as interventional modalities that have as much power in healing as the clinical medicinal interventions we are familiar with.

It does not matter which God you believe in or what religion you practice. Spirituality has been shown to improve all illness parameters in all people. Carl Jung said that his patients who believed in God and an afterlife did better with life-threatening illness than those who did not believe. He said that regardless of whether God existed or the afterlife or reincarnation were provable, simply having spiritual beliefs was clearly beneficial. Recent research at Duke University Center for Spirituality, Theology and Health, showed that elderly people who had any kind of spiritual practice, including church attendance, daily prayer, and meditation, had less chance of dying within five years than people with no spiritual life.

# Your Spiritual History

*This project opened my eyes to my spirituality. I had lost spirit and faith in God when I lost my family. Now it has been returned to me.*
— **Christine**, Spirituality and Creativity in Healthcare,
University of Florida

This week our goal is to tell the story of our own spiritual history. Art and healing illuminate your spirit, so your spiritual journey shines bright and true.

Artistically speaking, your spiritual journey is a life work. Whether you're a nurse, artist, counselor, gardener, engineer, or doctor, this week is about opening up your spirituality to interface with your whole life. If you are connected to your spirit and follow your calling—what you truly long to do in life—your work will be given in service with reciprocal joy as a perfect expression of who you are as a full human being.

Your life has been a pilgrimage to get to this moment in your creativity and caring. You bring with you the lifetime of your ancestors. Their lifetimes and spiritual journeys are present in your life in this moment and present for those who will share it with you. You're not here by accident. You made a conscious choice to pick up this book and start the journey inward to heal. Now is the time for your spiritual transformation.

What is your spiritual history? What got you here? Think about your ancestral ties and upbringing. Most of us have attended a church, mosque, ashram, or other temple. More and more, people are finding the many benefits of yoga, meditation, guided imagery, and other methods of relaxation.

As we start to dig into this week, you will enlarge the sacred space in your life. This will deeply honor your spiritual work and amplify the intelligence of your heart. This work will allow you to intentionally make art that is healing within your own sacred space.

## *Resonating with Your Spiritual DNA*

A spiritual thread ties us to our ancestors. It is buried in a microscopic strand of nucleotides: our DNA, a massive parade of humanity. The thread is a long string of other lifetimes, fused together in a tight helix that morphs through time as the ancestral pattern repeats and modifies itself when we are born and continues after we die.

"Spiritual DNA" is a new term used by health futurists to refer to how your body carries your ancestral spirit. An ancestor who lived five generations ago, for example, is represented by DNA inside you. You may not be aware of this person, though they are present in your genetic code. Part of your art-healing work is becoming conscious of the possibility of unconscious imprints from the past. When you summon your ancestors, they know what's in your body; they know about things and events that you may not.

We are largely built from DNA that goes all the way back to animals. Our bodies immediately react with physiological changes to ancient images and sounds. The sacred space of ceremony and dance is a transformational door. We are built to resonate with certain sounds—with dance and drumming ceremonies, for example. When we experience them, we heal deeply from the past. When we change inside, we change our outer selves as well. Then we experience healing transformation in a higher dimension, far beyond where science can go.

## Finding the Sacred in Your DNA

The earth is constantly changing and evolving. We become conscious of that as we make art to heal ourselves, others, and the earth. There are also ancestor spirits who share our DNA—they literally live in our bodies and share their stories of past lifetimes. Part of our work honors the wisdom of our ancestors and fulfills our ancestors' destinies as their descendants. Your grandmother dreamed past the limits of her life's journey. She birthed a child, continuing her spiritual line. You are part of her destiny. We fulfill ourselves and our life journeys when we honor our ancestors' lives and our past lives. You have an incredible opportunity to fulfill your ancestors' destiny. You can liberate them in this lifetime.

In this work, we will make an intentional connection to ourselves and the earth. As you move through spirals of transformation, your axis is like the earth's axis. You are part of a constellation; you live in a body connected to your journey in the star clusters we live in. Part of your work is to be deeply connected to earth energy, because when you tap into earth energy, you tap into natural creativity inherent everywhere.

The first step is to ground yourself in your body. Mastery of your body lends insight, allowing deep, inherited patterns in your DNA to manifest. Some patterns may not have been lived; they need to be born and transformed. When you do this process, you feel your grandmothers' and grandfathers' paths in this lifetime. You will call on family and friends to be part of your sacred community. Their spirit serves you in this work. Your past relationships will inform and heal you in the present moment.

## Reclaiming the Divine Feminine

Part of reconnecting is to embrace the divine feminine, the mother in us all, creator, nurturer, lover, giver, and receiver. She is the embodiment of holding and embracing. She is the container for the growth of life. She is the generous womb that creates the forms of our dreams, holding and nourishing them until they are ready to be born. The divine feminine also holds aspects that are irrational, nonlinear, emotional, and vulnerable.

When we merge with the divine feminine, we have an opportunity to merge with the part of ourselves that is nurturing, generous, sustaining, and receptive. The feminine is an aspect of humanity that has been long suppressed and disempowered. When we tap into art as a way of healing, we encourage the reemergence of the divine feminine.

In ancient times it was different. Some of the first healing and transformative art is about the divine feminine. Neolithic sculptures used for ceremonies in Europe showed a large woman with big breasts and a round belly. Petroglyphs found all over the earth show the divine feminine and women in ceremony. Cycladic Greek sculptures showed women with arms upraised, as if performing a ceremony. Ancient sites in Greece were consecrated with the divine feminine worship; the first statues were women with arms upraised. In Chartres Cathedral in France there is a cave with a sculpture of the Black Virgin. The sculpture portrays the dark, unknown feminine. The Black Virgin is a goddess who destroys illusions and what's not working so that new things can be born. She gives birth to death. Kali, another divine feminine figure, is the Hindu Goddess of empowerment. She is a goddess of time, death, and change. Her consort, Shiva, is made of light. She is the ferocious form of the mother goddess.

There are so many women in the field of art and healing that art and healing truly make the divine feminine visible. Jean Watson, a nursing theorist and scholar who founded the Watson Caring Science Institute, brings the divine feminine back to nursing with her emphasis on caring. Rachel Remen, MD, with Commonweal, is bringing the divine feminine back to physicians and medical training with her emphasis on emotions and art. Since this work is the embodiment of divine feminine energy, the women who practice it are seen. This is a crucial part of art and healing. One of the reasons we talk about the divine feminine is that allopathic medicine has been dominated by the masculine. Science, technology, linear thinking, and other masculine aspects dominate our culture, society, institutions, and humanity. We address the radiance of the divine feminine to return to the aspect of ourselves that is creative, erratic, irrational, emotional, and caring.

To be open and creative, you need to allow what seems "irrational" to be expressed so it can be seen, heard, and embraced. Art does not need to make sense. You don't have to understand or explain what you make. This is a process that does not have to make sense and can be irrational. Give yourself permission. Just be with it.

When you make art to heal, you bring the divine feminine back into your body and bring this way of caring back to your life. This is an important part of how Art as a Healing Force works. The divine feminine is a necessary part of caring, loving, and healing. In Chinese medicine, feminine yin energy is nurturing healing energy; masculine yang energy is action-oriented healing energy. Modern Western medicine has put yin energy to sleep. Science has taken over, displacing nurturing with technology.

## Marrying the Divine Feminine with the Divine Masculine

In addition to losing our cultural connection to the divine feminine, we have also lost the concept of the divine masculine. In our culture, the masculine is often portrayed as violent, materialistic, domineering, and destructive. In fact, the divine masculine is about penetration, seed, energy, light, creation, trance, healing, and inner travel. In ancient times, the divine masculine was completely different. For example, Apollo, the Greek god of the sun, was the god of music, oracular power, consciousness, medicine, and light. The divine masculine is much different than the "masculine" stereotypes we talk about today.

Art and healing gives us an opportunity to reunite the divine feminine and the divine masculine within ourselves and create an experience of wholeness and personal integration.

Many cultures had a sacred marriage of the divine feminine and divine masculine as an important basis of ceremony. Many earth sculptures showed the two mating. The *Hieros Gamos*, or sacred marriage, was important in Sumer, Egypt, and ancient Greece. The island of Delos in Greece was the birthplace of the twins Artemis, goddess of the moon, and Apollo, and is an important place where these two energies merge. Bee priestesses, or Melissas, led ceremonies in ancient Greece to celebrate the union of the divine feminine and divine masculine. Followers of Dionysus had sexual ceremonies for the union of energy. Tantra in India and Tibet unites the divine feminine and divine masculine to achieve enlightenment. These images, paintings, sculptures, dances, and ceremonies are deeply healing. They bring opposites together and merge them as one.

When you make art combining the divine feminine and divine masculine, you resonate oneness in your inner artist-healer. The process allows both masculine and feminine aspects inside you to fall in love with each other. This is a manifestation of the ancient Spirit Lovers, a sacred marriage of the first lovers in human history, myth, and legend that represents the birth of all things. Both halves are inside everyone. When they are recognized, they bring wholeness to our soul. Our art-healing groups are attended mostly by women. Most of our university workshop students are women. The few men who come are beautiful. They are discovering the feminine part of themselves. When women see their feminine side and men learn to see women as the divine feminine, everyone falls in love. This is deeply integrating and healing for both the women and the men. Art and healing are one, like lovers.

Art and healing bring the divine feminine back to healthcare. When the artists come into a hospital (or heal themselves) with dance, beauty, music, and poetry, the divine feminine muse returns. The divine feminine seduces the spirit to dance with her, and a magical integration takes place. The divine feminine and the divine masculine merge, and a magical collaboration takes place that is nothing less than spiritual and healing.

## Laura's Story: The Moon Goddess Heals

When we bring art into healing, we tap into feminine ways of knowing, which means caring, not fixing. The masculine is about curing symptoms, but art as a way of healing is about caring, nurturing, and loving. The divine feminine energy is essential, not complementary. This divine feminine aspect is critical if we are to be in balance in the way we heal. Any interventional action model needs to be balanced with receptivity and nurturing as well as allow for the invisible and unconscious. The emergence of feminine energy (goddess energy) balances the whole healthcare system. The emergence of the Goddess within your life gives voice to Hygeia, the Greek goddess of healing.

Recall week 2's story, in which Laura told about healing herself from rape with dance. In making her dance, she used many spiritual tools. She invoked the Goddess and spirit animals. This was valuable to her healing process. She told us,

The difference between what I decided to do for this project and what I've done in the past was that I set very clear intentions for my work. I also chose to use guided imagery and drawing as other tools in the process. I created an altar in my room next to the space where I dance. I would light a candle, burn some incense, and sit to do the guided imagery.

I began by just intuitively creating imagery for myself. I brought myself to a safe space and began to visualize a warm, healing light pouring over my body. Eventually I added the visualization of the chakras and the colors and seed sounds of each one, focusing on the second and fourth chakras. I would then visualize my spirit guides, ancestors, angels, and spirit animals surrounding me, connected to me. I felt their protective presence and reassured myself that I am constantly being guided and protected.

I would then close the imagery by chanting or singing. I drew pictures and put on music that I loved, and danced. I began to see a pattern in the pictures I started to draw. I felt very connected to the image of the Moon Goddess, so I drew a series of Moon Goddesses. I began to add in the chakras when I drew her.

When Laura danced to heal herself from the trauma of rape, the Moon Goddess danced inside her. Laura was led to an art-healing experience that was more beautiful than we could ever have imagined.

## Week 3 Praxis

This week's praxis is all about becoming aware of your spiritual journey and of the pilgrimage that is your life. This is a time in the Art as a Healing Force program to take time to write in your journal. You have had a whole life up to now, whether it's been sixteen, thirty, or seventy years. You have a spiritual evolutionary experience that is your own life story. You have parents who came from your grandparents. You are a spiritual being having a physical experience in this life. This praxis is an opportunity to review your life as a pilgrimage in your journal. Tell your story.

Your writing is a reflection to deepen your ability to feel, see, and remember your own spiritual life journey. In this exercise and in your writing time, invite the presence of people who have come before you, giving you this life. Feel your connection to them, if it's appropriate. As you live your life, realize that one day you will give your life to the children of the future.

Take out your journal and write your spiritual history. Tell the story of your spiritual life, from childhood to now. Write your spiritual history any way you want to—as a story, myth, timeline, or history in prose. When you feel moved to write, spend this week journaling about your spiritual life, how it started, what you did, and what you do now. You can write about important events, practices people, teachers, and retreats. Invite memories of the most important spiritual moments of your life. See, feel, and relive them.

To help you along, here are three Medicine Art projects to infuse more spirituality into your own art-healing process:

- Find your healing muse
- Discover your spirit animal
- Make a medicine wheel

## *Guided Imagery: Meeting Your Healing Spirit Muse and Guide*

A spirit guide is a presence in your life that feels like a beloved ancestor, religious figure, or angel who watches over you and protects you. It's a palpable presence that many people experience as love, a higher consciousness, or even God's embrace. In many different spiritual traditions, gods and goddesses represent human emanations and energies that are part of all humanity. Gods and goddesses represented their different emotions and actions and are guides. For example, Tara in Buddhism is caring. The Hindu Kali is destruction, rage, and creation. Many people we work with receive images of spirit guides when they do their Medicine Art and draw, paint, and write about these experiences. Images of figures of healing and power come to people and are an essential part of art and healing.

Standing in this place of freedom, focus on the area around your heart, expanding your field of love as if it were an enlarging bubble. Allow this feeling to radiate from your heart to your head, down your arms, and through every cell of your body. As you focus on this feeling, awaken your healing muse, which will guide you through the rest of this twelve-week journey.

The muse inspires the artist and may even send images or ideas to help make the art. The muse helps the art-making process be something wonderful. Your muse can be someone who loves you deeply, who would happily hang your art on their wall, who would play your music or dance with you, and who understands that what you are doing is beautiful.

The muse of art and healing is more than a muse to just make art. They inspire you to make art to heal yourself, others, your community, or the earth. The muse sends you healing images from beyond ordinary life.

As you focus on this feeling, imagine the person—a past relative, teacher, or figure in your life—who supported you and your art. Bring these images more clearly into your consciousness, feeling the love they have for you and the love you feel for them opening in your heart like a flower blooming. Maybe you can see a grandmother, a great-grandmother who has passed, a spirit guide, or angel. It could be a friend, lover, ancestor, religious figure, revered teacher, or a new presence in your life. You can even invoke someone beyond your own lifetime, blessing you from some other time and space. See a figure or energy who knows exactly who you are. Your muse knows what you are supposed to do in this lifetime and breathes creativity into you as you make art. Feel the muse loving, blessing, encouraging, and praising you as you make something truly beautiful and healing for you and others.

Invite your spirit muse to be with you and guide you as you make art. Imagine your spirit muse telling you how wonderful you are and how the art is healing for you, someone else, and the universe. When you're creating art with the intent to heal, it helps to picture in your mind's eye your healing muse and your loved ones in your life while you create. Invite your muse into your inner workshop or studio. Let them fill this place with inspiring ideas and images for you. Let them love you, support you, and tell you that you are doing exactly the right thing as you make your healing art project.

### Medicine Art: Draw from Guided Imagery about Your Healing Spirit Muse and Guide

In your journal, write about the experience of what you saw when you were imagining your inner spirit guide. Who were they? What did they look like? What is your guide's connection to you?

For the people in our classes, the muses vary. Each person has a different muse. One woman's muse is her grandmother, whom she's never met. The muse stands behind her and strokes her hair as she paints. For others, the muse is an artist-healer guide, like Alex Grey or Christiane Corbat. When we go around a circle and ask each person to describe her or his spirit muse, what we hear from people is mind-blowing.

## *Guided Imagery: Meeting Your Spirit Animal*

Spirit animals are wonderful opportunities to have an animal's essence and wisdom come to you. Spirit animals are protectors, teachers, and guides. They lend us their wisdom from their natural way of being in the world. Throughout human history, our companions are all the animals that lived or died. When you call in spirit animals, you have opportunities to honor your animal body, since your body has DNA that comes from animals. Many artist healers use spirit animals to bring up the ancient energy in the spiritual DNA of the animal's powers. For example, you can call on lioness energy to bring the powerful energy of the lioness into your life. Shamanic healers would not work without spirit animals accompanying and protecting them. Spirit animals are portrayed in art in shamanic cultures to share the experience of visionary healing.

This week is one of the most exciting weeks in our twelve-week program. When we do the Art as a Healing Force process with people, they very much enjoy getting a spirit animal. It has become an important part of many people's art and healing process. For example, Anna Halprin, cofounder of the Tamalpa Institute, an expressive arts teacher, and the grandmother of healing dance, teaches cancer patients to dance with their spirit animal to get strength and courage. This guided imagery will help you meet your spirit or power animal. Spirit animals come from deep within human consciousness and are our deepest memories. In the memory of our very cells, we can see out of a lion's eyes. We are the animals. This guided imagery exercise can be done to connect with your spirit animals.

Close your eyes. Take a couple of deep breaths, letting your abdomen rise and fall. Go into your imagery space as you have before. Let your breathing slow down and feel your body relax deeply. Now imagine yourself standing on a path. Feel your feet touch the earth, smell the fresh air, and feel the warm breeze on your face. Feel the ground and the soil as you walk down the path. Smell the grass on each side of the path. Let the path lead you to a place you love in nature. It can be a meadow, a mountain, or a forest. Sit down in this beautiful place and rest. Enjoy the sweet-scented air and see the sunlight.

Now ask your spirit animal to come to you. Pause. Allow for anything—any image—to emerge slowly. Be patient and calm. If you don't see an animal now, don't worry or feel pressure. It will come later or another day. Look all around you in this magic space. Let the animal appear and come up to you. Don't censor or analyze the animal that comes. Simply accept what you sense is there.

The animal may come from a distance or appear right next to you. The animal looks like an ordinary animal coming out of the mist. It may appear suddenly or slowly. The animal that appears to you is your spirit animal helper. It may begin to speak to you in an inner voice that sounds like a thought but feels like it is not yours alone. You can ask your spirit animal a question, such as why they have come to you and what they will help you do. You can speak to them and tell them what you want. Spirit animals may not speak in words; they may speak in riddles or feelings. Tell your spirit animal you will visit them, feed them, speak to them, and be with them.

You can stay in the beautiful place as long as you wish. Your spirit animal is part of the earth. It has tendrils that reach deep into the earth, the sky, and you, connecting them all together. If you feel comfortable, let the animal touch you or even come into your body. You can merge with your animal and see out of its eyes.

When you are ready to leave, say good-bye to your spirit animal, stand up, and leave the place. Walk farther down the path. It leads to the edge of a forest of old-growth trees. Stand at the edge of the forest. Find a tree that beckons you. Put your hand on the tree and touch its rough back. Feel its warmth, its life. Now imagine that when you put your hand on this ancient tree, you move deep into the spiral of your own being. You spiral deep inside yourself, into your heart, and inside your body. Your heart opens like wings. A spirit eye within you sees this experience. It witnesses your journey.

Slowly come back to the room where you are. Bring your spirit animal with you. Bring your sense of connectedness with you. Move your feet. Look around you. You are now on the art and healing path. You can see and hear your spirit animal's voice telling you how to heal the earth. Each time you talk to your spirit animal, they will be more accessible to you. If you don't talk to them, they may rest in the distance and wait. If you have T-shirts, small toys, or sculptures featuring your animal, you can bring the animal closer into your consciousness.

The spirit animals are the wisdom keepers of the earth's energy and magic. When we see out of the eyes of the animals, we hear the wisdom that resonates within them about the earth's energy. We hear how to be in balance and harmony with the earth. This is everyone's birthright.

## Medicine Art: Draw, Write, Dance, or Sing Your Spirit Animal

An important part of art and healing for many people is drawing, painting, writing, dancing, or singing your spirit animal. When you make art after your guided imagery to meet a spirit animal, the memory and information you saw will deepen your experience. A lot of the art made in our twelve-week process deals with spirit animals because they resonate with our spiritual DNA. For this week's extra project, you can make spirit animal art. You can draw, paint, or collage; you can also make jewelry, a T-shirt, or a dance, or write a journal entry. Do anything you want to do. Making art with your spirit animal will invite the animal to be more powerful in your life.

## Samantha's Story: Meeting Her Spirit Owl

Samantha's wonderful and emotional journey of art and healing was profound and beautiful. Each week she made art—sometimes furiously—to heal her trauma. One week she learned that her spirit animals were life-changing and necessary on her journey to heal herself with art. She told us,

> In addition to all the visual art and writing I did, I had another deeply life-changing experience through this art-making process. For a period of about two weeks in late October, I had a very strange series of dreams. In these dreams, I saw an owl in the trees above me in a dark forest. Sometimes the dreams were frightening, but somehow I knew that the owl was there to help me through this darkness and find a new pathway to light.
>
> She and I never spoke but communicated in other ways. She would sweep up above my head so that her feathers would touch my face. I would become her in the trees and felt her wisdom in me. I felt as if her patterned wings were my arms. I felt wind underneath me and floating and flying sensations. In these

dreams, I also saw a woman who seemed to be an ancestor of mine. She was old and looked very wise, in a weathered way. Her wrinkled eyes with crow's feet at their corners seemed to say so much about her. She was brave and strong and had a sense of concern for me, as if she were worried if I would find my way. I began to see her in the trees as well and became strongly aware of my personal connection to trees through these dreams.

Samantha drew, painted, and made jewelry each week about her owl to help her and protect her as she healed from trauma.

## *Medicine Art: Making a Medicine Wheel*

An alternative praxis for this week is to make a simple medicine wheel. The medicine wheel was used in many ancient cultures. It was like a compass in spiritual space, used to orient people to spiritual energies. It was also a calendar that aligned people to astral energies. It was a time indicator for the seasons, related to astrology and the sky. Sunrise in the east represented new beginnings; sunset in the west represented healing. Medicine wheels were a way that people found their center. We use the medicine wheel in our Art as a Healing Force program to make a sacred space. It is like an altar; it protects people and helps bring in healing presences to make art.

To make your own medicine wheel,

1. Draw a circle.
2. Draw a cross in the circle, from east to west and north to south.
   - In each direction you will ask for a different energy to come to your life.
   - East represents new beginnings—what you are beginning in your life.
   - South is the manifestation of your passion—your art, drawing, and writing.
   - West represents healing, dreams, and the unconscious mind.
   - North stands for grounding and wisdom.
   - The center is Spirit, whether it's Mother Earth, Father Sky, God, the Virgin Mary, or another figure from any religion or spiritual practice.

Now find objects that are meaningful to you in your life. They can be religious icons, animal carvings, feathers, stones, jewelry, pictures, a gift from someone you love, or anything that is sacred to you in your life. If you want to use spirit animals, you can do the guided imagery exercise to help you find the animal who chooses you, or you can simply let an animal call to you or attract you when you look in one of the four directions. Place your sacred object in the direction that it symbolizes for you. For example, you could place a gift from your partner in the south, for love.

Start by putting your hand down in the east. Think about new beginnings, change, the wind, air, and young children. Let your sacred object call to you and put it in the east.

Now move your hand to the south. Think about passion, manifestation, falling in love, energy, fire, and youth. Let another object call to you and put it in the south.

Move your hand to the west. Think about healing, power, water, deep dreams, inner spaces, and adulthood. Let an object for healing call to you. Put it in the west.

Now move your hand to the north. Think about wisdom, grounding, family, work, what makes you feel safe, elders, and the earth. Let an object for wisdom call to you and put it in the north.

Now put your hand in the center of the circle. The center is your life. Think about your spiritual center. Reflect on who helps you and guides you. Let a figure or an animal call to you. Put it in the center.

You have made your first medicine wheel. Close your eyes, bless your medicine wheel, and ask it to change your life. Say you will make a medicine wheel again. Leave in peace.

 Michael shows how to use a medicine wheel to create sacred space. http://www.youtube.com/watch?v=ejk1uQp2fIM&list=PLMm-0ccB -CYpmKktLEws7WlrNyNg2QDnu&index=12

## Troy's Story: Ten-Minute Daily Spiritual Practice

Spiritual practice is an art process. In combination, art and healing allow us to experience a spiritual space. Many people who did the Art as a Healing Force program chose one spiritual practice, and they did it during the twelve weeks, along with making art, journaling, and creating their final project. They found that a daily practice deepened the work and kept them calm and grounded as they healed.

Troy was a student in her last year of college. She was getting a BA in religion but did not know what to do when she graduated. Her path in life was not clear to her. When she came to class the first week, she had just broken up with her boyfriend and was grieving the loss of an important relationship. Troy used a daily spiritual practice as part of her art and healing work.

> Along with journaling each week, my praxis included making art daily and weekly and working on my final Medicine Art project. I practiced yoga every morning with the intention of blessings and gratitude. I also attended a yoga class once each week and painted at least once each week. My painting would be meditative. I used watercolors and just allowed myself to paint whatever I wanted.
>
> As I started bringing sacred space into my daily life, the rhythm of my life began to change. The painting would calm me. While I created, I could feel the flow of the watercolors and the brush on the paper. It was a space to be with myself more than a time to do art. My yoga time set the tone for my days, and as the twelve weeks continued, I started to feel very blessed and grateful.

After graduation, Troy kept art and healing in her life. She continues to make art, practice yoga, paint, and heal. She now lives in Northern California and is part of a thriving young adult spiritual community. She completed a Yoga Teacher certification and lives in close touch with her soul daily.

At the end of this week, you are invited to do a spiritual practice. You can:

- Transform space in your daily life to be present and creative
- Find examples of spiritual practice that are opening to your own creativity, such as meditation, yoga, guided imagery, and prayer
- Do a personal spiritual ritual, like lighting a candle and praying
- Burn incense on your altar
- Listen to special music
- Engage in yoga or body work
- Listen to guided imagery or meditation
- Do ten minutes of drawing, reading poetry, or writing poetry
- Stretch or do healing movements
- Do self-massage
- Practice tai chi

- Play a musical instrument
- Write letters or poems to someone you love
- Make a flower arrangement
- Make origami
- Sing a song
- Read a spiritual book

All these practices open your heart and deepen your spirit to make healing art. It is important to realize this when you do the spiritual practice. It is quality time for yourself.

## Summary of Week 3

- Write your spiritual history in your journal.
- Embrace your healing muse and spirit guide with guided imagery.
- Do the extra guided imagery to meet your spirit animal.
- Draw or make art about your new spirit guides and spirit animals.
- Try creating your own medicine wheel.
- Begin a daily spiritual practice.

# WEEK 4

# FINDING OUT WHAT
# NEEDS TO BE HEALED

*There is a story within us that longs to be told, a poem within us that longs
to be spoken, a dance within us that longs to be stepped, an image within us
that longs to be seen. Allow the mystery to emerge from within.*

Welcome to the fourth week of Art as a Healing Force. This week is powerful.
We will take you deeper and begin to address what you need to heal in your life.
Using art as a healing force is a transformative experience that heals you at the core of
your being. It goes to the core of your life and uses guided imagery and Medicine Art to
get to your needs, pain, and suffering.

Let's engage the artist-healer within to find what needs to be healed in your life.
You will now look deeper to see what needs to be attended to and what needs to be
healed. You can bring this aspect of yourself into the creation of an artistic life. It can
be in yourself, others, your community, or the earth. You may need to heal from a physical illness, mental condition, or spiritual growth issue in yourself. You can heal other
people, such as a brother who is ill or people in hospital programs; create healing in the
environment, a river, or a mountain; or heal anything that calls to you.

You may have a unique, personal story of pain and suffering. If you don't have such
a story, you may be carrying suffering from others in the community or in the world.
Many people feel alone in the darkness, have sadness in their life, or endure suffering.

Your pain may be hard to understand in the beginning. This is an important step when you take this journey to heal.

Darkness is the three-dimensional place where pain resides. How do we honor pain and suffering we have experienced? How do we own our story? This week is an opportunity for you to remember your story, hold it, and transform it into a creative healing journey. You can transform your suffering into art with our creative process. Take what has been injured and hold your experience in your hand. By telling your story, you are holding pain in a sacred way to honor pain, suffering, and darkness. Look deeply at your story of darkness this week and transform it into light.

As we approach our pain and suffering, we will hold it and engage it in a physical way with art. With dance, painting, poetry, music, and ceremony, we take an energetic place that may be stuck and move it into a new way of being. This creates liberation and a deeper understanding of self. The creative process releases you from your pain and deepens your experience of humanness and understanding. As we heal what is wounded inside, the healing of the wound makes us strong. The journey of the wounded healer makes the shaman.

Finding out what needs inner healing requires speaking from your heart and being able to authentically listen to its voice. The Art as a Healing Force process is about illuminating and sharing your healing need from within.

**What Needs to Be Healed**
- What are the gifts of your life that you have not given yourself, received, or acknowledged?
- Do you have feelings that have been pushed aside?
- How does this affect you?
- What do you know about this deep challenge you hold within?

Whatever your healing need is, the world has it as well. Your healing need can be addressed with your own creativity as an offering for yourself and others. The best service to the world is to bring light to your own healing need. As you listen to yourself, tell your story, and listen with your heart, your witness within emerges. As you listen to yourself, be heart-centered. Do not let your thoughts be pulled into the drama of your story. This is not about "fixing." When you listen, be neutral, reside in the still point of your heart and life, appreciate yourself, and make a loving connection.

Let's step back for a moment. This is an opportunity to engage with the core of your own being. What is your purpose? Why are you here? In your personal journey, set the intention of informing and transforming your core consciousness.

Your healing art is an opportunity to simply reflect on your own life. What is most important to you? What is your gift that you can see when you go to your essence to heal? Allow this project, this journey, to be an opening for the re-patterning of your own life. As you use your creativity intentionally for healing, you are re-patterning the whole. This re-patterning is for your entire life. It goes beyond the physical body. It is an energetic re-patterning of your entire perception of life—more than the objective world as you see it. In this field of being, we are re-patterning your entire human being. As a human being, you are not an object; you are a subjective, spiritual, whole being. Everything you do to and with your body you do with your whole being.

Your art and healing work is to realize your wholeness as you re-create yourself from your heart and your soul and restore the profound nature of your love and creativity. This process is about creating a connectedness to yourself. Within you, a divine creativity sustains and organizes your life. Your journey is about increasing your awareness of this powerful connection with your own higher consciousness.

In this process, your creativity develops your own ability to understand and share your experience with the world. All human beings belong to each other. You reside in an infinite field of divine love. Your creativity can open up channels that put you in right relationship with the universal divine source of creativity. In the still point of our being, we have access to the channels for healing. Open up to this spaciousness that is incomprehensible; it is the heart source of all humanity. In this place, there is an exquisite calmness, a dignified composure. You are able to witness your soul without ego. Who are you as a spirit-filled person? Seek to see yourself with your heart's eyes, seeing yourself with beauty, dignity, and positive regard, honoring your very own humanness.

How do you do this? Your thoughts create powerful energy. You can heal by simply being who you are in a creative moment and allowing your thoughts, feelings, and body to express what needs to be healed. In your creativity, which is the expression of your soul, you access the power of healing by simply allowing everything to be as it is. This is the beauty of the creative process and why it is so powerful for self-healing. Your own creativity offers an experience of reflection and engagement with your deepest healing needs. It allows for the opening of the natural outpouring of your heart.

Take some time to identify your own healing needs. They could be physical, emotional, or spiritual. They may occur in every aspect of your life. They could belong to you, others, your community, or the earth. *What really needs healing?* It could be as straightforward as a health condition. Ask yourself, *What needs to be healed? How is this illness affecting my life?* Begin by writing in your journal. We invite you to be open and honest. Just let your words flow. Write any unsaid words, both positive and negative, about your own healing needs. Write about the energies you hold in your body, dissonances in your mind, and your anxiety, judgments, and frustrations.

## Week 4 Praxis

Make a special space for yourself. In your mind's eye, create an area of protection. Build a completely safe place where you can journey inside yourself. We will start at the beginning to heal your experience of pain, sadness, or suffering.

As we go into this guided imagery, it's important for you to honor where you are. You may feel or glimpse nothing or something may emerge spontaneously. We will begin by simply focusing on the area around your heart. Breathe into the heart area. Focus on being centered. Gently inhale, filling your entire body with your breath. You are safe. As you do this work, remember that you are not alone. It's also important to remember that at this moment in time, you are perfectly capable, strong, and secure. No harm will come to you. Allow your memories to serve you. Everything that emerges in this guided imagery is there for your greatest good.

### Guided Imagery: Finding What Needs to Be Healed

Sit down, take a deep breath, and let go of tension. Feel relaxation rising from your toes and through your feet, calves, pelvis, and whole chest. Pause to feel your heart's energy expanding like ripples in a pond. Feel yourself soften. Feel your neck, eyes, shoulders, and forehead soften and relax.

Hold your body in your mind's eye. Your body speaks your life story. Ask yourself, What calls to be healed in this moment? Pause, deepening the experience of silence and spaciousness. As thoughts or feelings emerge, take notice. Observe the fluidity of your mind. Engage your sensory experience of your body. Ask your body, What part of me needs to be healed?

Whatever thoughts or images come up, allow them to emerge. Hold them for a moment; then let them flow away. Do not attach to them. Trust that what comes to you is right for this moment.

As your body opens, look into your darkness. You may experience a moment of pain, fear, contraction, or not wanting to hurt. Hold that emotion. What does your dark place say? What does it look and feel like?

Your are witnessing this experience in sacred space. Go deeper into the darkness. You may see yourself as a child. You may see yourself being frightened, or you may remember a moment of being in physical pain. You have already lived through this experience. This is only your beginning. Let your story take form and unravel what has been locked and held deeply inside you.

Now imagine in your mind's eye a golden thread. Hand it to the hurt part of yourself. Your inner witness holds the thread and says, "My intention is to remember you, hold you, and heal you." With the golden thread, connect the part of yourself that's hurt to the part that is strong, capable, creative, and wise. This is the beginning of the creative connection to heal this part of your body from the darkness.

Slowly come back to the room where you are. Feel your body's contact with the chair or floor. Experience your weight and physical form. You are back in your body. You are whole, well, and ready to begin to heal your darkness by making art.

Mary talks about the process of finding out what needs to be healed and what you are passionate about.
http://www.youtube.com/watch?v=CaAPKksyKfs&list=PLMm-0ccB
-CYpmKktLEws7WlrNyNg2QDnu&index=11

## *Medicine Art: Draw from Your Guided Imagery about What Needs to Be Healed*

The powerful guided imagery we just experienced may have brought out images of what you need to heal. For your first Medicine Art project in this week's praxis, take out your journal or a large piece of paper and draw one of the images you saw. Don't be afraid. You are completely safe in this moment. Your journal will take your image and turn it into healing art.

# Samantha's Story: Painting Meaning into Life

Samantha was a sophomore in college when she took our class. She was an excellent student, with amazing energy to actualize what she believed in. She did not know anything about art and healing, and in the first week she came alive, like a volcano erupting. It was as though she were waking up from a long sleep. She opened her eyes.

For my Art as Healing project, I asked myself the question, What do I feel needs to be healed? When I sat with this question and meditated on it, I was astonished at how many things came up for me. I thought immediately of our earth, but many more things flooded my mind. I recognized so many things in my own life, my family's life's, my intimate relationships, my friendships, my city, my community, my country, and our Mother Earth that truly need healing. I often have a strong urge to help and to be a nurturer, so the task of choosing only one thing to heal for this project took some time.

One thing that helped me define this project was an experience I had during a guided imagery to find areas in my life and past that needed healing. I went to a place in my past that I had repressed in my memory for many years. During the meditation, I was catapulted into a flashback of being sexually assaulted by a man in the bathroom of a hotel room when I was fourteen. I was there, exactly in the same scene, young, vulnerable, scared, and alone. The images were frightening, yet re-experiencing this memory in my mind was somehow innately different than how it had happened to me the first time. This time I felt that some sort of guiding presence or protector that I had never sensed was with me before. It made the whole experience a little warmer and slightly easier to cope with. I came out of the meditation knowing that I wanted to address my past and my own wounds, especially the one I had just been reminded of.

After this experience, I invested a lot of time into writing in my journal and exploring all that was interesting and meaningful for me. I looked deeply into owls (which often accompanied me in my guided imagery) and what it means to have an owl as a spirit animal guide. I questioned what I needed to "let go" of in my life or what is no longer of service to me. I started to ask myself what I really want in my life right now and what I really need for my health and happiness. I started to verbalize my emotional states in my journal and understand them and myself more deeply. As the questions and writing kept flowing in my journal, my project became very clear to me.

Samantha has devoted much of her college life and career to art and healing. Now she volunteers as a bedside artist with Cindy Perlis in Art for Recovery at University of California, San Francisco Medical Center. She paints murals with healing intention. She works with pregnant women to help them de-stress and have healthy pregnancies. She has taught empowering art workshops for women, led art and healing days at her university, and worked as Michael's teaching assistant for several years. She completed a research project on how the Art as a Healing Force process heals, which will be part of her thesis. Her work in art and healing is ongoing, strong, and empowering to her and anyone around her.

### *Medicine Art: Journaling What You Want to Heal and Your Final Medicine Art Project*

Remember, the final Medicine Art project uses art—any art—to heal something in yourself, another person, your community, or the earth. This project should be something you will love doing. Imagine something you've always wanted to do but have never given yourself permission or time to do. This is the time to do it, whatever it is. It is time to create.

In the Art as a Healing Force process you will do it now, not in ten years. Ask yourself if you have ever wanted to learn to sing, make a film, or build furniture. If you can find something you're naturally drawn to, something you love and are passionate about, it will return you to the artistic part of yourself—what you've always wanted to be.

This book will support you in doing that, with the added intention of making art to heal. You will experience fully how creativity brings new life, energy, and healing into your life. You can start by simply noticing beauty. Slow down. Move from worry to being present in the moment; from fear of illness to beginning to heal.

Remember, you can do anything. You can commit to writing in the morning every day and become an author. Or you can become a photographer with your iPhone and Instagram or even a belly dancer.

Spend the next weeks with this question in the back of your mind: *If I could do anything I wanted to, what would it be?* Then do it. Do not worry or set yourself up for failure. Just by beginning, creativity unplugs the wellspring. Most people who have completed the Art as a Healing Force process say that they'd never thought they could do it. When you just start, anything can happen. During these twelve weeks, invite your inner artist to emerge. Don't worry about healing; that will come. Once creativity flows effortlessly, you will use it to heal.

To clarify what you want to heal for your final Medicine Art project, answer these questions in your journal. Answer the questions one at a time. Trust what you write, and remember to let your Inner Critic go.

- Where did you grow up? What was your family like?
- What is your major in school? What is your career path? Why did you choose it?
- What are your relationships like?
- What do you love? What is a hobby or art interest you may have given up as you made the life you have now?
- What are your goals? What do you want to do with your life?
- If you could do anything you want, what would it be?

Now pause. In this moment, feel our love and support as well as the caring of your art-healing group.

- Is there something in your life you want to heal?

Write in your journal the ideas that come to you. Don't censor them. Remember, you can change your ideas at any time.

Next, take your ideas about what needs to be healed and turn them into practical concerns for your final Medicine Art project. This may take longer as you think about what you want to heal and what art media you will use. In your journal exercise, be as specific as you can without limiting yourself. Be realistic—and for the fun of it, be unrealistic. Take it a step further. How does your idea align with what you long for—your deepest desire? Make a plan that involves a time frame, number of days, and materials.

## Make a Plan
- Prepare a timeline for your final Medicine Art project.
- Commit to the timeline.
- Get access to the materials you'll need.

- Commit to a time of day or a day each week when you will work.
- Identify resources you need to do the project you envision.
- Get involved in the creative process.
- Identify people whose help you need for your project.

Write all this down in your journal slowly, working from your heart or from the voices of your inner guides. Write your truths as though you are speaking to us.

When you do this, you create a relationship with who you are. Hear yourself speak about yourself. Experience your own story and see the significant events in your life. See your life path, your job, and what you gave up to be where you are now. Find your dream for yourself and see something in your life you want to heal.

Next week, go back in your journal and read what you have written and rewrite it. As you rewrite it, let the story invoke deep feelings. Rewrite until you get a sense of what the connections and compelling themes are. What keeps coming up? What is filled with energy? What do you resonate with? What makes you buzz and vibrate when you read your answers? Make your story alive by using words that evoke emotion so that a reader can be in your shoes and see out of your eyes.

At this point in this book, it is essential to identify your personal intention to heal a specific aspect of your life. When you create an intention clearly and focus on it, the healing need can speak to you. This requires all your senses. Part of focusing like this is identifying your healing need, feeling it, allowing yourself to embrace it, and merging it into the flow of each chapter's creative processes and your final Medicine Art project.

## Laura's Story: Freeing Herself through Dances

We've been following Laura, Michael's past student at the Institute for Holistic Health Studies at San Francisco State University. She told us more about using dance to heal the trauma of rape and how this process helped her find meaning in life.

In the guided imagery I did to try to see what elements of my life needed to be healed, it was very clear to me that I needed to focus on healing myself from the trauma of being raped. I kept this part of myself quiet for ten years, and recently, I have been working on it in different ways. In my guided imagery, I understood that it was very apparent that it was still affecting my relationship with myself, the friends I made, and my boyfriend.

Initially, I wanted to create not only a self-healing project but also a project that I could bring into the community. I wanted to try to use my project as a way to help other women regain their power and feel a sense of closure. But as I began my work, it was clear that I needed to focus on my own healing before I could help anyone else.

Dance has always been my way of connecting to my body. It was something I discovered after I was raped. I remember having the realization that through movement I had broken down the massive wall that separated my mind and body. That was years ago. Since then, dance has served as a sort of spiritual connectedness and grounding.

Eventually, through improvisation, I somewhat completed a dance that I performed. I feel very good about this process. I feel as if I have relived the struggle of breaking free, and I have created enough that I no longer feel those chains. Eventually, I will take this to the community and I will help others move from the destructive, disempowered place that I am all too familiar with.

Thank you for the encouragement to face those demons and for facilitating a safe space in which to explore all these elements. It was truly life changing!

A week after doing the dance that completed her Art as a Healing Force program, Laura got pregnant. Now she is a mother and married (to her boyfriend), and has a whole new life. Laura's dance freed her body to become a mother.

## *Other Examples of Projects for Inspiration*

People who have done the Art as a Healing Force process have created thousands of projects using visual art, music, dance, words, or ceremony to heal. We will be providing a much more detailed list of instructions and examples of final projects, but these are some examples to help you develop an idea of what you want to ultimately do for your own final project:

- Sewing a quilt to heal chronic stomach pain
- Making a painting to deal with leaving a childhood home
- Dancing to heal a mother after the father has left
- Building a huge circle of stones on a beach with family as a memorial service for a grandmother who passed

- Making a painting to heal a relationship with parents
- Performing a ceremony to grieve for a lost pregnancy
- Cleaning a river's banks in prayer
- Listening to stories of border crossings and making poems that will empower immigrants
- Performing a ceremony with visual art and dance to heal a daughter's breakup
- Performing a large ceremony with poetry and dance to heal a whole family from a death of a grandmother who had never been properly grieved
- Performing a ceremony with narrative and costume to heal a daughter's menarche
- Leading a guided imagery and using visual arts to heal a brother with a brain tumor
- Making paintings to heal cancer
- Creating an empowerment dance to heal a rape
- Making a bracelet to heal memories of childhood sexual abuse

## Kylie's Story: Her Final Medicine Art Project

Kylie was a student in the Art and Transformation program at John F. Kennedy University. For her final Medicine Art project, she chose to concentrate not on herself but her community. She worked in her own unique way. She told us about her final Medicine Art project.

Nothing inside me was crying to be healed, so I decided to send my love and art out to the community to do some healing. My partner grew up in Southern California, and all through his childhood, he visited the convalescent homes where his mother worked. I decided that I wanted to bring a plethora of art materials for the residents to play with during an art-making session. I wanted to be able to encourage them to feel their innate creativity and be free. I wanted them to find new ways of experiencing and expressing their thoughts, memories, and world. I hoped that I could let all this be felt.

I began by writing a letter to the administrator at the home, introducing myself, expressing my beliefs around transformative arts and my intentions of employing art as a healing power. She invited us to visit and told us that they currently did not have any art supplies or funding for art materials.

We arrived, set up, and began the relationship before the art materials were introduced. This was helpful because during this time, I learned that group-guided imagery would not be appropriate, considering the observable cognitive levels and attention spans of many of the residents. I chose to abandon that plan and to simply show them how to use the materials and invite them to create whatever they wanted to. Approaching a blank paper with endless options was a challenge for many of the residents. Gentle encouragement helped them overcome their fears about ruining the blank paper or beliefs that they are not artists. It was lovely to watch them become more comfortable with a paintbrush; spectacular to observe their awe about the colors washing across the paper; and sweet to see their amazement over the concept of a rubber stamp. It was completely fulfilling to witness it all.

Since the art-making session was so effective, I am now confident that I am capable of bringing art into the community and creating an impact . . . I am grateful for my blessings that allow me to share my passion for creativity with the residents at the convalescent home.

Kylie plans to develop a nonprofit youth arts activism program where children can select a topic that concerns them, research it thoroughly, and then create art to speak about their concerns. She envisions art providing youth with another voice to speak to the greater community.

You can choose anything or anyone to heal, with any media and any action. From experience, we know yours will be completely different—maybe even surprising to you. Every final medicine art product is different, each a gift of who you are in your authentic self.

This work is for *you*. It is not like a school assignment or project at your job. It will not be graded, judged, evaluated, analyzed, criticized, or compared to others. It will be received with love and grace, a gift of your beauty and honor. This is the process of art and healing. You are a powerful artist-healer. Your inner healer and artist are one. You can heal seven generations back and forward, as Native Americans say. You can change your world, your community, and even the earth.

## Summary of Week 4

- Do the guided imagery to find out what needs to be healed.
- Draw, paint, or dance from the guided imagery.
- Do the journal exercise to see what needs to be healed.
- Do the journal exercise to begin to think about your final Medicine Art project.

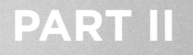

# PART II

# CREATIVE HEALING
## *WITH* VISUAL ARTS, WORDS, MUSIC, *AND* DANCE

# Creative Healing with Visual Arts, Words, Music, and Dance

In this second part, we focus on exploring the four main types of art media you can use to heal yourself, others, your community, or the earth. These next few weeks will also help you explore what you can do for your final Medicine Art project.

- *Visual arts*: painting, drawing, photography, sculpture, filmmaking
- *Words*: poetry, prose, drama, scripts, short stories, novels
- *Music*: Listening to music, playing music, singing, drumming, chanting mantras, using Tibetan singing bowls
- *Dance*: dance, choreography, yoga, tai chi

Each week, we'll be learning about and making art in each media by

- Finding and exploring images that heal with the help of guided imagery
- Making your own healing art from the guided imagery
- Learning more from the process by writing in your journal

You may find yourself leaning toward one medium or the other. You may already know what medium you'll use for your final Medicine Art project. Doing the process of making art to heal with different media will expand your knowledge and build new skills. The spirit of healing with art, as we teach in this book, invites you to open yourself fully to the possibility of creativity. Get excited to try new things!

We originally learned this from artists-in-residence in hospitals, who are open to using all kinds of media. They work with visual arts, words, music, or dance, depending on what the patient wants to do. Being open will expand your ability to heal with art immensely. It's also fun. You may even discover something that you'd never thought you would love.

# WEEK 5

# HEALING WITH VISUAL ARTS

*May we hold our hearts with tenderness and grace as we use art to heal
in the week ahead. May we align ourselves in mind, heart, body, and soul,
letting the innate wisdom of our mind's eye emerge and bear witness to the
deepest, most profound expression of our spirit. May we have faith as we open
our hearts and minds to the grand mystery within.*

This week, we would like to invite you to embrace your inner visual artist to harness the healing force within you. Each visual art piece you make this week will be a step forward in your healing journey.

Visual imagery is a powerful art form that over the ages has become more and more ubiquitous in our modern lives and culture—from glossy magazines to tablets, from the billboards by the highway to video footage played on the nightly news. This week is about concentrating on using visual arts as a healing modality.

Historically, many cultures throughout the world have used visual arts as a healing force. For example, indigenous cultures had carvings of spirit animals that were used in healing ceremonies. Christian art depicting Mary and Jesus is in every church, and Buddhist thangkas of healing Tara are placed in many Buddhist shrines. For centuries, Navajo sand painters and Tibetan mandala painters alike have been cultivating the art of creating images to deliberately bring about a change in consciousness and to promote healing and hope. Their art was believed to embody power.

A Maori carver in New Zealand told us this story:

I was making a huge Maori statue for a village. The statue was of a healing spirit, and I made it to protect and heal the village. A man came up to me and asked me the story of the spirit. I told him that the figure was a powerful warrior chief ancestor and that he would protect the village and help it heal. He asked me if it could protect and heal someone who did not know the story. I told him, "You don't need to know anything. The carving has power by itself to heal you and protect the village. The spirit comes down and lives in the carving and heals you from within it. The carving carries the healing spirit and his power." When I carve, the spirit carves through me. I just move my hands and it comes out.

Visual arts, in other words, have the power to impart ancient wisdom and sacred visions as well as to educate people to see more deeply. In Tibet art keeps wisdom and bliss alive and transmits it to others. Mandalas made in meditation by healing artists communicate balance, spirit, and healing. Colorful thangkas of healing depicting Tara, the goddess of compassion, are believed to bring healing and long life to the viewer. In this vein we invite you in the week ahead to make healing visual art that is focused on facilitating your own transformation, growth, or healing.

In teaching our classes over the years, we've found that visual arts are a good place to start for most people because they're so accessible. In fact, most people who use art to heal use one of the visual arts as a primary form of expression. When we say "visual arts," we mean a number of different media, whether it's painting something you saw in your guided imagery, sculpting a spirit animal out of clay, or drawing sequential art about your own healing story.

As we move into the praxis for the week, we will use two methods for making visual art:

1. The first method is free and spontaneous. Simply let your hands move. Draw a line or paint a color; then change, add, or erase. For this method, you do not have to think of a specific image to replicate. Let it come intuitively as you move your hand and fingers. Your body and imagination know what they're doing, so trust in them.

2. The second method is to access your mind's eye, see an image, and sketch or paint what you saw. You can sit peacefully, focus your mind's eye, do guided

imagery, or meditate—whatever produces a mental image you can copy with your chosen tool.

Alex Grey, the visionary artist who created *Sacred Mirrors*, finds the ethereal transcendental imagery in his paintings by envisioning it in his mind's eye first. He looks at it from all angles and then wakes up and re-creates it on the canvas. Other artists let their painting emerge from the blank canvas as it comes to them; their inner artist is guided by their body, imagination, and spontaneity. We invite you to experiment with both methods. Any combination of the two gets us to the same place.

Finding subjects for visual arts is easy. It's as simple as looking around you and borrowing from the world we sometimes take for granted. You may be inspired by myths, legends, and fables of other cultures and weave them into your own story. This process will happen naturally because these myths are in your spiritual DNA. You will see them during guided imagery.

### Artist-Healer Profile: Alex Grey—Visionary Painting

Alex Grey is a leading visionary artist of our time and a powerful spiritual leader. His unique series of twenty-one life-size paintings, *Sacred Mirrors*, takes you on a journey through your divine nature by examining, in detail, the body, mind, and spirit.

*Sacred Mirrors* presents the physical and subtle anatomy of an individual in the context of cosmic, biological, and technological evolution. Begun in 1979, the series took ten years to complete. During this period, Alex developed depictions of the human body that "x-ray" the multiple layers of reality and reveal the interplay of anatomical and spiritual forces.

After painting *Sacred Mirrors*, he applied this multidimensional perspective to human experiences like praying, meditating, kissing, copulating, pregnancy, birth, nursing, and death. Alex's recent work explores the subject of consciousness from the perspective of "universal beings" whose bodies are grids of fire, eyes, and infinite galactic swirls. Alex's work is an example of taking inner visions outward as art to heal yourself, others, community, or the earth.

Alex and his wife, Allyson, have installed *Sacred Mirrors* in the Chapel of Sacred Mirrors (CoSM), a sanctuary for seeing ourselves, the world, and our cosmos as reflections of the Divine. CoSM's mission is to build a temple to preserve and share a collection of visionary art for the global community. Forty acres of beautiful woods and buildings invite the contemplation of art and nature and provide a center for events encouraging the creative spirit. CoSM honors the mystic core of love that unites all wisdom traditions and the transformative power of art to awaken human potential.

Visual art as a healing force will help you "see" more deeply. When you make a drawing or complete a sculpture, you create images that did not exist before. Ancient and universal mythological images appear in visual art as you draw. Spirit animals, angels, guides, and ancestors appear. Remember that indigenous cultures used visual arts to share shamanic visions so that the tribe could experience and participate in the visions and learn.

To show you what we mean, here's a story from Michael. After being a facilitator to thousands of participants in the Art as a Healing Force program, he found himself in a place where he had to confront a negative prognosis. In this place of darkness, he found a way to make the art-healing process work for him.

## Michael's Story: Sculpting the Cancer Away

Both Mary and I have had many intense personal experiences of healing with art. One particularly art-healing event in my life happened long after I cofounded and taught Art as a Healing Force. It all started several years ago. I was driving to the airport to fly to New York. I was going to meet my literary agent and dear friend Alex Grey, and his wife, Allyson. As I drove down the interstate, I felt some discomfort in my back. During the two-hour trip to the airport, the discomfort turned into an excruciating, unbearable pain. Unable to drive any more, I stopped at a regional hospital, suspecting that it was most likely a kidney stone attack and that I would need some pain medicine.

In the ER, they treated me with painkillers and did a CT scan to see if the kidney stone had passed. The doctor came into my room afterwards and told me, "Your stone has passed, but you have a mass in your right kidney. You need to follow up on this." I was shocked. As a physician, I knew what a "mass" in my kidney meant. In one second, I entered the altered state of consciousness of a person told that they have a serious health problem. It was entirely different to take care of people who are sick than being sick myself. This presented a challenge for me that was as new as it would be for anyone faced with cancer.

I left the hospital. I was not in pain after the kidney stone passed, so I continued my trip to New York. While I was there, I worked with a woman rabbi who did healing. The whole visit was very difficult. I was worried and afraid but did things that were also deeply healing. When I got home, I got another CT scan. This one showed I had a mass in each kidney. The doctor told me, "This is probably lung cancer, metastasized to both of your kidneys." I knew I needed more tests and who knows what—surgery, chemotherapy, and more. In less than a week, my life had gotten very dark. I was plunged into the darkness of newly diagnosed cancer, a place I knew well from my patients, having been a physician artist-healer for so long. However, I had never experienced this darkness in my body firsthand.

An MRI showed a clear mass in one kidney and no lung cancer, so the prognosis improved from lung cancer, metastasized to kidneys, to kidney cancer. I chose a surgeon and hospital. The surgeon was the chaired professor of urology and a world expert on kidney cancer. He told me that the MRI definitely showed that I had kidney cancer and that he would remove the tumor and leave the kidney. They had to open my ribs from the back. It would be a long and difficult surgery with a hard recovery. I went home still reeling. My life had completely changed in one week. I went from seeing patients, doing workshops, and teaching art and healing to having kidney cancer and needing a painful, difficult surgery. I was upset, depressed, and afraid for my future.

*What would I do for three weeks?* I thought. I knew that I needed to do something to prepare for this sudden life-changing event, for my surgery itself, and for what would happen after. I had been working with cancer patients with guided imagery and art for years and knew most of the people in the alternative cancer community. I had a lot of support, a wonderful family, and people who loved me. My social support was covered, but I would still have to address the other slices of my healing pie.

Each day I simply followed my heart. I walked, grounded myself in my house and garden, and did guided imagery exercises to relax and see what I needed to do to heal my cancer and prepare for this surgery. As I did the guided imagery, delving into my dreams and my visions, I became much more positive about my life and optimistic about the future. I could see more clearly what was going on around me. It was as if the guided imagery opened my eyes and a kind of spaciousness appeared.

One day, in the guided imagery, I realized that I wanted to spend my healing time carving marble. Though it had taken me a bit to figure out, sculpting made a lot of sense, as I had been a marble carver when I lived in Greece in the summers. I loved the touch of soft stone, the sounds of the tools, and the visions I had when I carved in Greece. I had never carved where I live in San Francisco, so I found a piece of marble, bought carving tools, and found a sacred place to carve. The work of setting up a studio was exciting and stimulating. Just this preparation took me far away from cancer and surgery. I went from being in the darkness of a newly diagnosed cancer (the first theme in Spirit Body Healing) to going elsewhere in a place where I made art (the second step). My life force was awakening again.

My guided imagery fired me up with passion, and I started having visions of the spirit bears of the North. As a bear dancer-healer with Native Americans, the bear image did not surprise me. Bear was my spirit animal. I knew him well. But the polar bear images were new. I became obsessed, spending long hours looking at beautiful books on Inuit bear carvings, bears from Greenland, and bears made by Zuni Indians. My whole day was consumed by bear sculptures, images of bears, and the art of bears. This was the beginning of art as a turning point for me (the third step in the Spirit Body Healing process). I had gone from worry about illness to making art manifesting a bear spirit animal.

Then I began to dive into the visual-art healing process by making a small clay model of a sitting bear and using that to start carving my white marble. Each day I took my hammer and chisels and worked for several hours on my marble bear, carving by hand without power tools. The more I took off the marble, the more I watched with wonder at what emerged. My sitting bear came out of the marble, and next, a surprise: a bear spirit behind him. The bear spirit emerged from my bear's back, looking right at me. He was beautiful. My sculpture was now a bear with a bear spirit, which is common in Greenland bear sculpture. It had become a bear spirit transformation piece, and for me, it was a gift from my bear spirit.

In my obsessed and excited state, I knew I needed to do more. In my guided imagery, I saw a kayak, so I researched and bought a kayak. With my kidney problems, I knew I could not lift a heavy boat, so I found a light Greenland-style wooden boat and started paddling with the sea lions on the Bolinas Lagoon. Eskimos hunted sea lions from kayaks; bears hunted sea lions. Each day I went into sea lion space to look them in the eye and speak to them, and they to me. They told me of Eskimo hunters, of the bears who hunted them, of their babies. I looked into their eyes and saw the world of animals and my connection with nature; I saw myself healing. Sea lion, a second spirit animal, appeared to protect and heal me on this journey. They were strong and powerful. I felt their power, and I became stronger.

Then one day, my marble bear gave birth. A small man appeared in the arms of the spirit bear, cradled like a baby, loved and cared for. The man was tiny compared to this huge healing bear spirit. When I saw him appear, I cried. I knew the man was me. I felt the enormous love and care from the bear, from the bear spirit, from the sea lions, from far-away ancestors. I was calm now, happy, and even ecstatic. I had almost forgotten about the kidney cancer and surgery. I knew then that I was ready.

I went to the hospital almost in a dream. As I prepared for the surgery, I was with bear, not with surgeons. When I awoke from surgery, I did not know where I was. When I remembered, I was happy to be alive. My older son came into the recovery room.

"Dad, did you hear the good news?" he asked. I could not imagine what it was, except that I was alive. "The surgeon told me that the tumor was very strange—not what he'd expected. He was surprised. He said it was not malignant. It was very rare; it was hard and was like a small rock. He had never seen anything like it."

The surgeon told me they would do the pathology and see what it was. He said I was okay and should not worry. I know the bear spirit had healed me. He had turned the tumor into a tiny marble sculpture.

### Lessons from Michael's Story

- Making art to heal sometimes starts with the darkness of a newly diagnosed illness, such as the fear of treatments, thoughts of dying, and so forth.
- Guided imagery will relax you, promote a positive attitude, and help you find imagery to make healing art.
- Making art is a process that takes you elsewhere, away from obsessed worry.
- The images that appear by themselves in the art are homeostatic, self-healing images.
- Spirit guides may appear—animals, spirits, angels, anything.
- There can be moments of sudden knowledge when you realize you are healed or ready.
- Miracles—unexpected results not explained by science—happen.

# Week 5 Praxis

*Pencils, papers, and my willingness to heal myself*
*were my powerful tools to heal my heart.*
—**Camilla**, Institute for Holistic Health Studies,
San Francisco State University

For this week's praxis, we will do a guided imagery to see the world through your inner visual artist's eyes and then use one of the visual arts to heal yourself, someone you know and love, your community, or the earth. If you are using visual arts for your final Medicine Art project, you can go wild this week and try different media forms: sculpture, painting, or jewelry. Many times visual artists taking our courses set the intention to make art to heal, rather than make it for exhibition. Try a new visual art media: painters might try sculpting, a photographer might pick up some watercolors, and so on.

## *Guided Imagery: Finding Your Inner Visual Artist*

Close your eyes and relax. Slow your breathing. Imagine yourself in a place of tremendous beauty. Experience the delight of your own being. Take a deep breath and feel the life force that resides within you. This energy is a creative force—it is life-giving, the source of love. Embrace yourself and see your own light. Now imagine in your mind's eye that this light resides within your heart. This inner place is the home of great wisdom, intuition, and deep knowing. The gifts of your creativity are held in the mystery of your own being.

In your mind's eye, experience yourself as an artist. The creation of your art is about illuminating the beauty within. You are an artist, and everything you do each day is an opportunity to be creative. You have an artist within who takes life from the essence of your heart. The Inner Artist feels from the heart and sees from the heart. Connecting with your heart is connecting with the source of your images and stories and healing.

Go back in your life to moments when you were making visual art. Find the most beautiful, passionate moments of creativity as you see your visual artist within. Feel, touch, see, and go deeply into the spiral of visual arts. What were you doing? Were you a photographer, a painter, or a sculptor? What was the spirit of your art making—a muse, an inspiration, a dream? See deeply into the moments of making visual art. Now see yourself creating visual arts in your in life again. What are you doing? What imagery emerges? Rest and see the visual art flowing from your open heart, from the higher consciousness you are connected to as your visual artist within.

Breathe and become centered at the still point inside yourself. From that place, listen to your voice from within that says, "I am an artist. I am creative. I am confident. I embrace my whole life as my artistry. The life within me is the source of my creativity. Being an artist is a natural process of creativity in my life."

## *Medicine Art: Illustrating What You Saw from Your Guided Imagery*

This week's assignment is to create a piece of visual art from what you experienced during the guided imagery—what images arose from deep within you, what you felt and experienced during your trip inward, and so forth. You can pick one image that stands out and re-create it. If you are not attracted to an image, go deeper. It can be as simple as drawing simple shapes or color washes and letting them lead you to healing art.

In both our classes, we have people draw, paint, and collage for an hour or so after the guided imagery. Using this book, we have a week, so you can do more if you wish. You could draw with colored pencils, if you like, paint a watercolor, or do something even more ambitious.

A lot of people like pasting together collages. All it takes are a few magazines, a glue stick, some art board, and a few favorite art supplies like markers or glitter. Connect with things you are visually drawn to. Draw or paste these images into your journal. Make new shapes and forms. Become familiar with your imagery and ways of portraying it. Be patient and nonjudgmental with yourself as you draw. Just concentrate on each stroke with all your attention. Take time in your busy day to make this art in your journal.

You can take it into other media if you want to as well. Think outside the box. You can use your smartphone's camera or an app like Instagram to log a visual art-healing diary. Or start your own Tumblr account or personal blog where you post all your weekly art in graphics with captions explaining the process. Like Michael did before he started sculpting, you could take some clay and mold a spirit animal figurine for your altar, or use some play dough to make an art-healing mojo of your spirit guide. You can use film, stone, or metal—anything to express the images that came to you in your guided imagery. You can make figures out of found materials or decorate a skateboard. Anything goes. There are no boundaries here.

As you make the first lines or start bending shapes in the clay, you go elsewhere, a place where healing images come to your artist-healer. You connect with the part of yourself that needs to be healed by allowing the art to express your pain and suffering as well as visions of beauty. In this way, the steps of healing yourself with visual arts are just as simple as making art.

During the process, do not analyze your images or try to figure them out. This is not therapy, not a diagnostic psychological approach to healing. You do not have to understand what is appearing. You don't have to interpret or figure out who the figures are or what the colors mean. Trust what is happening and continue to make art. Creating a space and having access to a variety of different materials allows a creative healing process to simply emerge. Trust us—it works. All you need is the intention to heal with art. A drawing made with intent to heal will heal.

When we see what people in our classes are working on, it's beyond wonderful. Each person's process is completely different. They make faces of ancestors, bright light, colors like the sun, arrows piercing hearts like valentines, spirit animals, and more. As we walk around and look at the magic of the emerging drawings and the artist-healers' intense concentration, we notice the great differences between people. One woman may immediately begin a detailed drawing of a goddess, spending time on the figure's hair. Another may sit as though in a dream, take a brush, and simply let color flow across the page. Another person may doodle little stick figures, forming groups and villages. It is all good.

When you begin to create, allow your images to become real and tangible. In the beginning, it may seem like scribbles, doodling, and random shapes and images. But it's much more than that. The art of spontaneous and free doodling is not only creative but beneficial and healthy as well. The doodles are the beginning of glimpsed healing visions, the first strokes of what will appear. Maybe they turn into an angel or an aura of healing energy or become the exact shape and color that will heal you from abstract space. Trust the process. Sculptor James Surls, who makes spirits out of huge logs, tells a story about a time when he was in school and the teachers yelled at him for staring out the window. Now he realizes that he was looking for spirits that appeared years later and became the healing images in his art. So your doodles are real work.

Thom, a student, talks about his discovery and process of painting healing portraits through the Art as a Healing Force program.
http://www.youtube.com/watch?v=rZHGTDXmBrM&list=PLMm-0ccB-CYpmKktLEws7WlrNyNg2QDnu&index=10

When you make visual art, your own wonderful source of images begins to come into play. The images that emerge are totally different and unique. Images can come from memories, your imagination, dreams, or visions. They can also come from elsewhere—the divine, spirit guides, angels, or God. You can deepen the process of making visual art by creating a ritual that is similar to meditation. Allow the imagery to flow as you go inward. Treat this art as making magic or miracles. Each new line on the page or scene in your movie is an act of perfect, exquisite creation. As you draw, trace, cut, copy, or paste, connect to your inner self and allow yourself to move freely. Trust the process. Let go. Let the art and creative energies begin to flow. It may seem simple, but the lines, the paintings, and the drawings are leading you somewhere. Give yourself space to allow the creative process to happen. Let the art lead you deeply into its forms. Simply witness the work that is taking place.

Also remember to let go of your Inner Critic and know that when you are making visual art, it is completely your own. You are the artist, and you can make no mistakes. You can erase a line or change colors. Allow your Inner Artist-Healer to lead you. You are regaining your freedom. Art is ideal for the healing process because there is a tremendous sense of empowerment and little stress; it can be a doorway to healing and the expression of your soul. You get to experience the joy of your own creative process. When you make art—even a doodle—you change your body's physiology. By concentrating and freeing self-balancing homeostatic healing images, you go from stress and arousal to a state of relaxation, tissue rebuilding, and healing.

**Artist-Healer Profile: Christiane Corbat—Healing Art as Transformative Art**
Christiane Corbat (1945–2006) was a sculptor who used visual art to heal. She was an artist-healer extraordinaire. She lived in Barrington, Rhode Island, was married to a psychiatrist, and had two grown daughters. On the surface, she looked like an ordinary person. But in fact she was a powerful contemporary shaman-healer. Physicians referred patients to her by word of mouth and through her community and workshops. Her art and healing process were both original and ancient. She listened to each patient's story, looked deeply into them, and asked questions: Who are you? What do you love? What do you desire most? Who are your helpers? This took people from sickness to spirituality, a process that brought back their souls. Christiane and her patients went into visionary space to see what they needed to be healed. She saw the transformation.

She then made a sculpture to manifest this vision, a casting of the person or a part of their body in plaster. She created a process of putting the sick person in a cocoon—a second skin. She guided them to another world. Then Christiane took the castings apart and sacredly dismembered them and reassembled them in a completely new, sacred way as a person who is whole, healed, and in beauty. The person could see themselves from inside and then turned around to look into their own face. Their soul was revealed, intensely alive, and vibrating with energy. The person saw themselves with compassion, love, and a much deeper understanding.

Christiane eventually transitioned from casting people for individual healing to casting people to heal the world in the Globalheart Project.

> As I sensed the tension of world conflict, I felt a deep need to use my art to reconnect us to our longing for peace. In a meditation that day, I asked myself how I might do this. Slowly my heart grew warm and began to expand. In my mind's eye, I saw the earth within it and felt the presence of many other people around me. Each of us had the globe within our hearts, but each of us was holding this globe in his or her own unique way. With excitement, I went to my studio that day to create this vision of the Globalheart into sculpture.

Christiane asked people, "What is the unique gesture of your longing for peace?" Then she cast the person with that gesture, finally assembling all the castings in a ceremony with music to heal the world. This is a wonderful example of how making art to heal yourself or another person expands to making art to heal the world.

Christiane's work was based on collaboration, to help people reconnect with whom they've always wanted to be. She worked with individuals or groups as they faced serious illness, personal crisis, or simply wished to explore who they are. She addressed images that sustain or block true desire through the body-casting process she developed over her long art-healing career.

Christiane was a true artist-healer with a sense of mastery. She created a piece of art to reflect perfection in and of itself. The sick person saw and felt the perfection, took it into their cells, and was deeply healed. Christiane used sculpture, made relationships, used therapeutic touch, and saw deeply in her intuitive mind's eye. She was an intentional artist-healer with the courage to invent her own process.

## Checklist: Healing with Visual Arts

### Starting on the Path

- Think about your method of expression. Popular methods in our classes are sculpture, painting, photography, film, collage, jewelry making, painting objects, and creating costumes for a ceremony.

- Give yourself time alone to let your own healing images emerge.
- Ask yourself questions: What do you see when you are with someone? What can you invent as an artist-healer that will change you and your world? What healing visual art tools are at your disposal?
- Encourage creative ideas to emerge as visual images. Say a prayer for divine creativity to flow through you for peace.
- Buy paints or materials that look like they would be fun to use.
- Make posters and flyers, and put your work out there.
- Use your journal not only for writing but also drawing every day.
- Make an artist's tote bag that makes it easy to carry your materials.
- Set a routine to make art every day.

## Deepening the Art-Healing Process

- Make art to heal every day.
- Pay attention to your images of darkness and light.
- Let your images emerge without censorship.
- Respond to the materials that capture your attention.
- Cultivate a vision of looking at the world.
- Hang your art in your place of work, car, or home and on your art-healing altar to transform reality.

## Using Visual Arts to Heal Another Person

If you want to work with another person with visual arts, you can do this in several ways.

- Start by making a relationship.
- See the person in beauty.
- Ask them if they want to make art with you. Collage or drawing with colored pencils are the easiest.
- Make art materials available to them and facilitate their wonderful process.
- Make an art bag to take with you when you visit them.
- You can make art for them if they can't. Draw them, paint them, and make a healing portrait about their life and story.
- Create a ceremony with art for them and hang art around their space, hospital room, and so forth.
- Everyone is an artist. Everyone is a healer. Everyone can do this.

**Transcendence**

- Feel the power of something greater coming through your art.
- Be compassionate with yourself.
- There are no mistakes—only opportunities.
- Experiment with different materials, shapes, and colors.
- Listen to music to relax while you work.
- Remember that art is a spiritual meditation.
- Look for images of light and beauty.
- You don't have to show your art to anyone; it's yours.

## Summary of Week 5

- Do the guided imagery to find your inner visual artist.
- Draw from your guided imagery of being a visual artist.
- If you want to work with visual arts, make a sketchbook, sculpture, tote bag, or other work of visual art.
- You can work with another person using visual art. Give them supplies and see them as beautiful.

# WEEK 6

# HEALING WITH WORDS

*May our words flow from our hearts with the essence of who we are.*
*May our words vibrate with healing wisdom from our higher consciousness.*
*As the words flow, may they expand our heart's presence in our lives*
*and these healing words for others around us.*

This week we invite you to let your healing words rush out like a river from the inward source—in the personal language that only you can speak, the one you use to live, breathe, and create. Whether you are penning a poem for your lover, journaling about your dreams or intentions, or writing your own healing scene to act out, allow yourself complete freedom and joy.

Be willing to explore within yourself. Go to a place connected to your essence, deeper than fleeting thoughts, which constantly shift and change. Writing reveals what is true at a deeper level than the spoken word. Let your written words take you to a place deeper inside where you tap into the core essence of who you are. As your words flow, they reveal your inner world speaking. The voice of your soul, the part of you that creates meaning and manifests direction in your life, tells you your own true story. When you connect to this inner voice, you can discover the power of your own magic. You will learn to develop a dialogue with yourself and begin to hear, think about, and look at yourself in new and creative ways. This creates movement and transformation in your life.

Words are powerful tools; they have the power to change the world. With words you can travel into a world of creativity, conjure distant memories, reveal undiscovered aspects of yourself, and manifest new realities. Words focused intentionally on healing create change both physically and psychologically; they have the potential to tap a deep wellspring of healing energy within you.

## The Story of Your Life

The way we use words shapes our reality. Each of us already has a story that frames our lives, tells us who we think we are, and dictates what we focus on. They are the words we use to explain our present worldview. For example, our story might be

I am successful.
I am a healthy person.
I am in love.
I am getting what I want in life.

Or it might be

I am never able to satisfy anyone around me.
I am sick.
I never have enough of what I want.
I feel like a victim.
I fail because I am hurt.
I can't love anyone.

Almost every word you say reveals the story of your life at that moment. Your thoughts and feelings create the actions of your life—that's the story you tell. You create your life in the same way you create art—by creating stories. People say, "I am in limbo. I can't act until something happens." Or they say, "I am fighting with my husband. We have never gotten along." By listening to your words, you can hear what needs to be healed. Examples of common stories from many people are

I fail because I was hurt as a child.
I can't get along with anyone.
I can never change—it's who I am.

I can't fall in love.

My partner does not see me.

I'm not talented enough.

But words can also be used to create the change you want in your life. "You can restore by re-storying," said John Graham-Pole, MD, cofounder with Mary of Shands Arts in Medicine at the University of Florida.

Re-storying your life has tremendous power. Your words have the power to manifest reality. There are three simple ways to re-story your life. The first is through being aware of the words you use; the second, by changing the way you experience things; and the third, by looking for visionary experiences.

## Awareness

The easiest way to change your story is to listen to the words you use to describe yourself and what is happening to you. Then invite new words to come from your Inner Healer that are healing, positive, and show trust. Re-storying your life with healing words is powerful and can be done every time you experience an event. By turning your words around, you can turn your life around. Positive words create positive stories. With words of affirmation and intention, you can create a healing and thriving reality. One simple example is, "I paid too much—I always do." Invite new words when you tell the story again to reveal a healing story: "I found exactly what I wanted."

Being aware of what you say and welcoming affirmative and healing words are not about denying anything. Your first words express your darkness; your new words are your art-healing process and express healing and change. Many of our life situations are based on verbal interpretations we have practiced over and over again. Like changing any habit, you begin with awareness and then practice. Gradually you will see how those changes affect your reality.

## Action

The second step involves consciously choosing the way you use words about your life. Words create your reality. Just as Tibetan thangka painters choose to paint a healing spiritual image—either the goddess Tara for healing or Kali for change—you choose your new healing words, re-create your story, and change reality. For example, if you look at your house and say, "I wish I were living in a bigger house; I am a failure," be aware of what you are saying. The next time look at your house—whatever its size or stature—and invite healing words to come as your new story. Say, "This house is perfect for me at this time in my life."

See the transition? When you hear your inner words describing what you see, you invite yourself to look at the situation in a positive way. You can write your words down after an experience and see what you have written. Then you can choose new words and see how your perspective has changed. Again, the first words may be the expression of your darkness and what you need to heal, but the second words come from your inner healer, describing your new reality.

## *Visionary Re-storying*

The third and most powerful way of re-storying your life is based on inviting a visionary experience to come to you. We use art and healing, guided imagery, healing visions, meditation, walks, prayer, vision quests, travel, and Medicine Art to reveal your visionary experiences to you. Having visionary experiences of inner guides, helpers, or angels is deeply healing. Our process promotes your imagination and visionary experience.

Afterward, we have people make art and write down their visionary experience in their journals. In this way, they can honor and receive it and make it part of their worldview. In peaceful moments, they hold the vision; in dark moments, they reach for it to comfort them. For example, if a person hears an inner spirit guide of their grandmother telling them they are beautiful, this inner voice becomes stronger and is more deeply felt.

Patients who use art and healing have experiences of angels, spirit guides, animals, and nature forms. Each visionary experience is used in re-storying. The person with visionary experiences and a spiritual life is a person with protectors or helpers in their life. We have found this to be profoundly healing for physical problems and life crises. This phenomenon of visions creating new stories is common and wonderful. A woman whose son died saw him come to her as she played music, and he told her how much he loved her. This was deeply healing and became her new story of his death, replacing the story of empty loss.

New research at MIT has shown that memories can be changed by substituting in new information. Memory, or the story we carry, depends on words and images. By replacing existing words with new words, you can actually change your memory of a traumatic experience to a memory of being loved. For example, a memory of being abused can be replaced with images of being loved by someone above. That love in images and words slowly replaces the previous image of trauma.

As the story of your life grows, you keep retelling it with new words and ways of seeing. You can make yourself the hero or heroine. One woman with breast cancer was making a garden to heal. Her story changed from being a depressed victim to a story in which she was a creative, powerful woman who was creating a fantastic mandala garden to heal. As your story forms, tell it, claim it, and take responsibility for it. As you change your language, you change the way you see and invite a visionary reality to come to you.

The most basic re-storying of our lives is accepting who we are as artist-healers. "I am an artist; I am a healer. The artist and healer in me are one. I heal myself with art. When I make art to heal, I change my life and the lives of all those around me." Re-storying changes our view of ourselves in a fundamental and powerful way. We move from seeing ourselves as someone who does not know what to do when faced with illness or crises (maybe someone who has been to many therapists and still is depressed) to someone who has the skills as an artist-healer to heal themselves, others, the community, or the earth.

Here are some other examples of re-storying your life by your words.

## Examples of Stories in Positivity and Love
- I can succeed in my work and relationships.
- I can see beauty around me.
- I am on the right path to becoming myself.
- I am learning from this and growing with each moment.
- I am being guided and taken care of.
- I am in the right place.
- I can love the people around me.
- I have always been loved.
- There are guardian angels around me who love me.
- My spirit guides have always been with me, taking care of me, and loving me.

## Affirmations to Help You Re-Story Your Life
- I have choices every moment.
- There is magnificence in action all around me.

- This is so beautiful.
- Love will heal me and those around me.
- This is meant to be.
- Each problem is a way to evolve and grow.
- My actions are guided by a greater force.

**Components of Healing**
- Self-love
- Forgiveness
- Being guided—you are not alone
- Choice in every moment
- Things come to you as gifts
- Seeing through the eyes of an artist
- Faith and trust
- Belief in God, angels, guardians, and spirits

In this week's praxis, we'll be doing various writing projects. As you work, keep in mind the power of the words and stories we tell you.

## Michael's Story: Healing with Words

My wife, Nancy, died of breast cancer in 1993. She was fifty years old. She coauthored many books with me, including *Well Pregnancy Book*, *Well Baby Book*, and *Seeing with the Mind's Eye*.

While my wife was having a bone marrow transplant for breast cancer, I wrote a journal about the experience, and it probably saved my life. I stayed in her room in the hospital for the five weeks of the procedure. Watching her undergo this difficult procedure and worrying about its complications was as hard as anything I had ever done. One part of me held the story that she could die—a real risk, they told us—or have terrible side effects and suffering. This was one story that I could have lived in and become depressed and ill.

But my inner artist emerged. I decided to bring a laptop into her room and write each day. I awakened to the world of my story and the world of her transplant. I found that each day, as I saw what was happening to her and to me, I would also see it out of my healing writer-artist eyes. I also saw her spirit and gave thanks for seeing it. Instead of being sad or being a crisis report, my journal became deeply spiritual. It became a story of bravery. Nancy was my teacher. Each time I wrote, I saw differently. I perceived what was happening to us in a way that was sustaining for me, not depressing. My vision was of her beauty, not her suffering. I hold that vision even to this day. And it was the writing that let me see this illuminated reality rather than just focusing on the incredible difficulty and darkness that was happening. This came through in the journal as well. It was always brightness and prayers of thanks that transported me out of the room to a place of vision. I think if I did not write, I would only have seen the darkness. With writing, I was able to cross a bridge into the light.

When Nancy was dying, we all suffered immensely. My older son dug a koi pond while his brother sat with her and played his guitar. I sat with her and watched her. There were two realities I could see and feel, two stories that were emerging in my life as the observer. One was her body, dying, yellow, bloated, and incontinent; the other was her immense beauty and the light that was around her.

As she went in and out of a coma the week before she died, she started to tell each person who came to visit that she loved them and that they looked beautiful. She looked into their eyes and rested in silence. To me, she was so brave. Her beauty far surpassed her physical situation, and the way her body looked was not what I saw. The love that flowed from her was a gift to everyone who came. Her love was visible and what I held on to. Elizabeth, her best friend, took me downstairs and said to me, "Michael, you know Nancy has shed her personality and become pure spirit. She is perfect love now, to be given to each of us." I knew this was true. I could see it and feel it.

This was the beginning of my re-storying of Nancy's death. I chose a new way to look at her, wrote a story to concentrate on, and worked to make it real. The new story became the source of my perceptions and created the reality I have today. I could see events that fit into my story of her death being transcendent.

My perception of Nancy's pure love and the light around her was what got me through her death. It was so bright for me that the whole process seemed like it took place in grace and in light. She had become pure love to be given to all of us. Compared to the power and immensity of what I saw, her death almost receded.

I told the story to people during her death and after her death. Later, I wrote a journal of Nancy's death with that story in it. Rachel Remen wrote about seeing Nancy's death as love in her book *Kitchen Table Wisdom*. With time, the story became real for me and for others. The story came from my new ways of looking at Nancy, my visionary experience, and Elizabeth's and Rachel's stories and experiences.

### From "Only Things of Beauty Persist,"
### Michael's Bone Marrow Journal

*April 1993*

We lay together before dawn like two children waiting for Christmas morning, excited, expectant, and nervous. We were also afraid, but our love tied us together; we were as one in God, awaiting the coming.

At dawn, I opened the drapes and let in the joyful morning sun. The human spirit is like the dawn. It comes up from the darkness, from nothingness, and floods the world with hope and joy. It dazzles and blinds us at first with its rays and reminds us that it is a new day.

The eucalyptus trees shimmered in the breeze, reflecting the green light of new life. I put a sacred Taizé chant on the tape deck and read Julian of Norwich to Nancy.

> I may make all things well, and I can make all things well, and I shall make all things well, and I will make all things well, and you will see yourself that every kind of thing will be well.
>
> You have restored my life, O God, and I wish to be in your presence.

I had showered and combed my newly cut hair and put on a dress shirt for the occasion. The sun shone into the family room where I got ready. It was like suiting up for an event, preparing for a wedding or bar mitzvah. The excitement filled the air like energy or electrons and made us both nervous. My body was shaking inside with tiny vibrations, like a taut rubber band. The nurse said that this was the long-awaited day, but the procedure was not much—just sucking the defrosted marrow into large syringes and pushing it into Nancy's central line.

At eight, a woman pushed a cart into the room and happily greeted Nancy. She said she was Joy and "here to give you back your bone marrow." She started to arrange the trays, water, and syringes. She poured water into the bath that would defrost the marrow. I plugged in the heater and motor to warm and gently shake the water. Smiling and telling Nancy not to worry, she called another nurse and took Nancy's marrow from a small ice chest and checked each of the five small flat bags to make sure that the name and number matched those on Nancy's wristband. She said that although it was a day filled with significance, the procedure would not hurt and was no different than putting something into her IV. I opened up my heart and prayed for her.

*Thank you, Great Spirit, for your world. Thank you for this dawn and this new day. Thank you for Nancy and her life. Thank you for the doctors and nurses who care for her and their love. Help her, Great Spirit. Help her live and get rid of her cancer. Give her a good life; let her be born again and be your child and be one with your world.*

I saw the light in the room change. I could see the molecules of air light up, an energy was visible that surrounded her and filled the whole room. It was like the light itself danced around her. The whole room was lit from within.

# Week 6 Praxis

The words you write are preludes to the words you speak and the actions you take. As we said earlier, be aware of the powerful resonance of your words. When you speak, you create a vibrational energy for yourself and your environment that interacts with the nervous systems of other people and resonates with their minds and bodies. When a word is spoken by many people many times and reaches a certain resonance, it can change physical reality. Similarly, when you say, "I love you," or put love into your actions or art, it is imbued with an energetic field that can change you and the whole world around you. The word is a force, a power.

Use your words as a force of energy to release yourself from what binds you and keeps you from being free to heal. In this week's praxis, we'll use words to do this in several powerful ways. The first is a free-association exercise in your journal, the second is writing poetry, and the third is writing a drama.

## *Free-Association Journal Exercise*

For this exercise, make an appointed time each day to write. You can write anything, from the musings of your soul to your daily to-do list. Mary makes small drawings and doodles in the side margin of her journal. The writing process is just a stream of consciousness; the idea is to simply let it flow. This is a process of pre-reflective writing with the words flowing, without pausing and thinking about them.

Give it a try. For your free-association entry in your journal, imagine that you are floating along on your stream of consciousness and don't know where it will take you.

When you begin to write, just allow the words to happen. They don't necessarily have to make any sense. Release your worries of grammar and punctuation and let words resonate from your heart. Open your inner spaciousness and give yourself permission to simply write. Let your words go beyond thinking and theory and be lived experience. You can write about your family, a dining room table, fresh flowers blossoming, or a simple message to begin your day. Write down the things you want to do or review the last ten years of your life.

Giving up control removes the obstacles of fear and criticism when you start writing, especially for people who don't think of themselves as writers. Let yourself be engaged in the words. Explore, play, and experiment. Ask yourself, *If I let myself play, what would I do? If I did not have to write something great, what would I write about?* There is no expertise necessary here. Do it your own way, following your natural inclinations. Make it fun. Spark your sense of adventure. You may like to write quickly and recklessly or slowly and carefully. You may like to write with tiny letters or big letters. Feel free to try different styles of writing and see what feels best to you. There is no wrong way—just let your natural style emerge.

If this exercise feels strange, awkward, irrational, ugly, childish, or repetitive, that's okay. The less you judge yourself, the more words will flow. Write about an event you experienced in your life. Choose new words with the intention to change your life. Choose your words with a new way of looking at yourself. Please respect and keep what you write, going with the feelings and following your energies. There are no guarantees, but the outcome may surprise you.

You can also write only one or two words on a journal page or on a blank page and make a drawing, painting, or collage about the words. This is powerful, and many painters use it as an art form. The written word focuses your energy like a lens, and the drawing or painting emerges in beautiful circles or spirals around the word.

## *Poetry and Healing*

Poetry is powerful. It is often more evocative than prose, since it works through imagery, emotion, and sensation, and is therefore closer to our right-brain image processing. Poetry is the language of the soul. It gets to the core of feelings and senses and comes from intuition. Poetry seduces you to go elsewhere; it creates a desire to reach out from your heart. It can be lyrical, mystical, and ethereal.

You can write about love, sadness, and pain. The more deeply you feel, the more beautiful your poetry will be. A glimpse into yourself reveals something greater than you knew you could feel. Words help you experience a new depth of knowing, feeling, and experiencing. It can feel like the words were messages from your inner muse or divinely sent from God. Like a mystery, your words reveal clues to a truth, emotion, or experience. The poem guides you to a place deeper than you have ever gone before. Once you write a poem, you are there. Just write. Feel it. Read it. Aren't you surprised by what you made? Poetry is used extensively to heal in hospitals and cancer centers and is part of the large vibrant field of poetry and healing. Rachel Remen uses poetry with cancer patients at Commonweal in Bolinas, California. In her preface to John Fox's book *Poetic Medicine* she wrote, "Poetry is simply speaking the truth, and one of the best kept secrets in this technologically oriented culture, is that simply speaking the truth heals."

### *Medicine Art: Projects to Heal with Words*

Take out your journal and write a poem or several poems. When you write, don't worry about rhyme, meter, or rules. Use them if you want to, but anything goes. Let it all come out. As the first line comes to you, let it write itself. Use words that evoke feelings, imagery, and experiences. Then, if you want to, you can read your poem out loud to yourself or share it with someone.

More simple words as healing projects to work with are:

- Write one word on a page in your journal and make a drawing about the word.

- Write poetry for one week. Get up each day and write a poem or do it at another time of day. Write anything. You don't have to show it to anyone.

- Get up every morning, get a poetry book, and read a poem. Find a book that you resonate with. Maybe it's a book of love poems by Rumi. Read, and then rewrite the poem in your own words. Feel as if you are the poet. Write in the first person, using "I" so you are fully there.

- Write a love poem. Look at the moon or a sunrise and write about it. Be with your beloved and write a poem to them. Write a poem to your mother, even if she has passed away.

## Keith's Story: Mourning Sickness

Keith Smith wrote this poem about dealing with his wife's death. Before her illness, he was a visual art teacher at a community college. He attended a cancer retreat at Commonweal and started writing poems there with Rachel Remen. Although he was an artist, he had never used his art to heal. When his wife died, he used journaling, poetry, and drawings to deal with her death. With this wonderful work, he became an artist-healer. He published a book, *Mourning Sickness*, with his drawings and poems. Here is a poem he wrote about healing himself from grief.

**"Mourning Sickness"**
mourning sickness
growth and change
dance this dance
with loss and pain
see the furred petaled and winged world
eating destroying being born and unfurled
searing fearful horrific and blind
peaceful potent serene and sublime
testing, testing
are you ready to conceive
to deal with
what is dealt
from the magician's sleeve
you are pregnant with God
you are great with soul
giving birth to yourself
is life's greatest goal
do not be stillborn again.

In this poem, Keith goes deeper into his healing. The animals come to him as guides. He sees images of birth and of his new life to come. Now Keith is married again and has children. His grief helped him give birth to his new life. Keith called his work "The art of grieving." Art and poetry are wonderful ways to heal grief for family and friends of people who have died.

## *Declarations of Love and Appreciation*

Poetry or a short powerful string of words is a good way to tell people how much they mean to you or how much you love them. This has powerful healing effects that ripple through that person, out to the world, and back to you as well.

One way to do this is to use your art and healing writing skills to write a vow, an oath, or a pledge. You can use creativity, healing, and love to write your own vows for a lover or a pledge to a friend. Open your heart and let your words flow. The vows need not be for a wedding; they can be for any ceremony or just for love.

Remember, when you write a poem, don't worry about rhyme or meter. Anything goes—it's about free emotion. Start with a first line, let the next one come to you, and watch it turn into a whole poem.

## *Using Drama to Heal*

Drama and theater are also deeply healing forms of using words. They have been used since before the ancient Greeks popularized the art. Theater re-creates real-life events or imagines fictional ones that embody power. People watching the drama can experience the events, learn, and be moved by them. This re-experiencing of events is deeply healing when done lovingly in a safe space. In a drama, the event becomes alive. The actors and audience live, embody, and taste the story; the images become real, affecting physiology. Theater can deal with emotion, things that happened, and imaginary events. When it has a powerful subject like rape or relationships between family members, both the actor and the audience experience the story and are healed by its coming into the light.

## Anita's Story: Saving Her Daughter from the Soldiers

Anita's job was doing theater with AIDS patients. She knew a lot about art and healing, since it was her daily work. She devoted her life to healing people with art. She came to Michael's class at the Institute for Holistic Health Studies to learn how to make her theater process deeper and make it more healing. She was a Latino woman and very beautiful and emotional. We watched her as she did her guided imagery about what needed to heal and saw tears in her eyes. We thought she was going to do a project about her wonderful AIDS theater, but when she presented we were surprised.

She brought her seven–year-old daughter and ten-year-old son to class. She put a small keyboard in front of her son. Her daughter was dressed in a beautiful Mexican flowered dress. She passed out beautifully painted paper butterflies she had made and gave one to each person in the class. Then she spoke.

> My family was from a small village in Mexico. Generations ago, the Spanish arrived and one night took away all the daughters. This story has been haunting me my whole life. My mother told it to me, and my grandmother told it to my mother. As I did the guided imagery, I knew I had to heal this story once and for all. My village had a butterfly grove where monarch butterflies came in migration. It was a beautiful village in the mountains. You could see the fog blow in, the tall trees, and the butterflies nesting with their wings slowly moving.

She laid her daughter on a soft mattress of eucalyptus leaves—the leaves the butterflies ate—while her son played a soft melody she had written on the keyboard. Then she did a dance. She circled the room, touched the butterflies in each of our hands, and brought us all to her village, centuries ago. As she touched them, we found ourselves moving the butterflies' wings. We could feel the wind and the soft wings of the butterflies on our faces as she danced around us.

Then she stood in front of her daughter. She was so strong. She looked the soldiers in the eye and told them they could not have her daughter. She lay over her daughter and protected her perfectly. She kissed her and stroked her face and enveloped her in a powerful blanket of pure love. Then they both stood up and danced together to the music her son played.

We could not believe what had happened. It was as if her daughter were saved from being kidnapped. Life was returned to her, to her family, and to the village in this beautiful dance.

### Lessons from Anita's Project

- Your project may not be exactly what you'd thought it would be when you started.
- You can heal generations in the past and old stories that haunt you.
- Family members can help.
- In art and healing, theater is healing ceremony.
- Make an environment, sets, costumes, music, and a script.
- Make a whole healing ceremony by combining visual arts, music, dance, and words.

- Theater excites emotions, involves the viewer, and heals them.
- Make theater from events in your past.
- Make theater from events in your own life.

### Guided Imagery: Making a Drama from a Painful Event in Your Life

Like Anita, you can create a short drama to return to a place in your life that needs to be healed by expressing and re-creating it in a healing way. You can make drama from a painful event in your memory. It can be dramatic or very soft. Be assured, you hold this experience in your body already, and with this creative process, you will be able to return to it and hold it from a new space and new perspective.

You may do this alone in a safe place, with a friend who can hold you in silence in a safe way, or in front of an art-healing group. For this drama piece, you will create a one-person play, and the lead character is you.

The guided imagery takes you to the place inside yourself that holds this memory. When you come back, you will create an improvisational drama where you embody the memory again. In the guided imagery, you may imagine other people in a three-dimensional place, such as a room. In your imagination, you can speak to the people who were present during your memory. The whole process takes less than five minutes. When you complete the improvisational memory play, sit down for another five minutes and breathe, feeling yourself embraced by love and seen by your own healing inner witness.

To begin the guided imagery, sit down or lie down and make yourself comfortable. Feel grounded in your body. Feel it in this moment in time. Feel yourself in the present moment. Remember the month, day, and year. Allow the chair or floor to completely support you as you move into your body. Now slowly breathe and count from ten to one, letting yourself relax more deeply as you count down. Breathe, saying a number with each breath: 10-9-8-7-6-5-4-3-2-1.

Release all tension as you breathe. Now imagine yourself in an open place of complete spaciousness. It is a safe place where you are calm and experience no harm. You are totally protected in this present moment. Settle into the still point of your own consciousness. In your mind's eye, remember a time in your life when something was painful. Return to that memory and see it like a film. Remember everything—the words, actions, feelings, thoughts, smells, age you were at that time, and physical location. As you hold this memory, feel the spaciousness of the present moment. You are in a safe place now, remembering this memory.

Hold this memory with love and compassion. Keep your body relaxed and hold the memory in silence. Be with this for a few moments until you feel the memory fade away. Now breathe. With each breath, count up from one to ten to emerge where you are safe in the present moment. With each breath, say a number: 1-2-3-4-5-6-7-8-9-10. Enter your body. Feel your feet on the ground in contact with the floor. Feel your fingers, toes, and your entire body in this present moment. Rest, holding the memory in your calm still point.

Return to your still point. Remember the present date and time to be grounded again. Experience the powerful energy you have enacted in your life. You have taken a memory from the past and released it into the present. This is your story. Let it go. Release it from your body. Feel your creative energy being released. Feel your heart opening. Release the memory with forgiveness. Hold the person you saw, and accept this part of yourself with deep gratitude. You have survived and are now strong and healed. Imagine yourself filling with deep gratitude and love. Now invoke a memory that brings you joy and love. This will infuse the old memory with light and understanding. Thank yourself for taking the time and courage to honor your own story.

These wounded parts of ourselves are part of our own humanity. In this moment, the past has been reconstructed and shifted into a new future. Step forward, take a deep breath, and be grateful for who you have become. In some way, you became who you are based on your own experience in this lifetime. It is part of your beauty and fullness as a person.

Now take three minutes to create an enactment where you will speak and dramatize the memory. This is improvisational theater. You can invite other characters. Open your eyes with consciousness, allowing yourself to embody the memory. As you embody it, remember that the incident has passed and you are safe. You have survived. You are strong, safe, and creative. You will re-create this memory and transform it. After you do the memory improvisation, return to your strong, safe still point. Now perform a three-minute drama of your experience, with other characters if they are there.

You can also make a small drama by speaking to another person as if they were your mother, father, sister, brother, child, wife, girlfriend, or boyfriend. For three minutes, look at them. Use your imagination to see them as your family member, and tell them what you want to say to them.

## Angela's Story: Sharing Life through Words

Angela was working as a nurse in a large hospital, and her life was very difficult. Her marriage was suffering from long hours at work. She was tense and anxious all the time. She felt her life was out of control and she needed a jump start to get it back. She told us her story of sharing her project.

I decided I would write about something very personal. I was in a process of self-discovery. I chose to write about my struggle to find myself, to find my own independence, and to grow up and take control of my own life. I wrote my autobiography. I described the hardships of leaving home, my fear, and my pain. As I wrote, I realized my life had been out of control. The more I wrote, the more I realized what so many people were trying to tell me. I had endured pain and trouble.

I never imagined that I would actually read it and share it with people. When I found myself opening up to share something so deeply personal, I could not stop writing. There was so much I wanted to share. I found that the process of writing allowed me to share. I did not have to share; it gave me the freedom to share. The most healing part was not just the writing but the sharing. It was not until this project that I was able to do something I felt really good about. By sharing I was able to touch the lives of others. I felt like my life was inspirational and my story could impact someone else. Being honest and letting others see my other side brought out deep emotion.

The class opened their hearts and minds and supported Angela in her growing processes. It was amazing how sharing with others allowed others to share with her. "I believe that I can incorporate how I use writing with my patients," she told us. "Many need to establish trust with their caregiver. I can achieve this by sharing, by allowing myself to be vulnerable."

### *How to Heal with Writing*

### Step One: Starting on the Path
- Be aware of the words you use in your life.
- Invite positive, caring words to appear and make new stories with them.

- Use the power of re-storying to change your life and move it in the direction you want to go.
- Take time to be with yourself to daydream.
- Create a space and a time to write.
- Value your writing time like it is gold.
- Use a laptop, desktop computer, spiral notebook, or journal.
- Make a notebook your portable studio and take it everywhere.
- Write every day for a set amount of time or number of pages.
- Invite your muse, wisdom within, or inner person of peace to sing to you every day.

**Step Two: The Journey of the Creative Person for Healing**
- Make an intention to heal with your writing.
- Publish, email, or blog.
- Share your voice; move out of yourself to community.
- Speak in public, to schools and churches, and among friends.
- If the whole page intimidates you, write in columns.
- Write small paragraphs or separate lines.
- Find colorful pens that delight you.
- Draw pictures alongside the words.
- Decorate your computer case or journal with beautiful pictures.
- When you write, let your words flow out.
- Don't edit or censor; let go of judgment.
- Write down what you would say to someone in words.
- Don't worry about making any sense at all.
- Feel love surrounding you.

**Step Three: Deepening**
- Write every day to heal.
- Jot down notes immediately when things come to mind.
- Bring symbols into your writing.
- Tell stories out loud to other people.
- Get into your stories; they will take you "elsewhere."

- Have conversations with your characters and invite them to appear.
- Allow yourself to flow on a river of words.
- Rewrite to make your writing more emotional and imagistic so someone can see through your eyes as you tell the story.

**Step Four: Transcendence**
- Tap into your inner wisdom and your soul's most powerful imagery. Put it into words.
- Poetry is often deeper and closer to the source.
- Find words in your writing that come up again and again; they are your themes.
- Love your words and yourself as you read them.
- Don't be afraid of poetry; you don't have to make it rhyme or have form.
- Create a support group to share what you've written.
- Bring out deep memories.
- Write a letter to yourself from your heart.
- Write a letter to the world from your heart.
- Let your words take you deep.
- Make your own life a living myth.
- Look for images of light and joy.

## Tips for Writing to Heal

- Be in the present moment.
- Write spontaneously.
- Write quickly, without thinking.
- Use imagistic words that create experience.
- Write from lived experience, not theory.
- Let your writing flow from your body and emotions.
- Write about whatever you feel like.
- Remove demands or expectations.
- Allow this time to write; move with the ebb and flow of your own words.
- Be comfortable in the silence.
- Be honest; both negative and positive expressions are powerful.
- Be authentic.

## Summary of Week 6

- Write poetry for half an hour or more and read it aloud.
- Do guided imagery for finding a drama in your life.
- Create an improvisational drama for yourself or others.
- Re-story something in your life and write about it in your journal.

All you need to do is write and the healing happens. It does not take much time, equipment, or space. You just need to make the decision to go into your writing place, write for a time, and then live.

# WEEK 7

# HEALING WITH MUSIC

*The sky and the stars make music to us; the sun and the moon praise us.*
*The Gods exalt us. The Goddesses sing to us. May our life flow with this primal*
*rhythm, song of the universe, and vibration of life. May our eyes, heart,*
*and ears be open to the music of this world and that which lies beyond.*

Music is one of the most ancient and powerful healing modalities. For centuries people have been using sound, toning, chanting, sacred songs, and drumming to put themselves into altered states of consciousness to heal.

Music evokes the spark of rhythmic, energetic engagement at the level of memory and emotion. There is clear evidence of a powerful healing force in music as a therapeutic intervention. Over the years and in many research studies, music has been studied in all health environments and has been shown to be effective for healing and symptom control. It is one of the most researched art media. There is strong evidence of the way music interacts with and molds the nervous system. Don Campbell's famous *Mozart Effect*, for example, showed that classical music helped children develop certain neurologic pathways, which led to increased cognitive skills and test scores. In another instance, music was used to increase mental alertness in the elderly. Many people unable to speak because of neurological damage have even been able to sing fluently after hearing music. Music opened neural pathways that facilitated language development and recovery.

Patients who listen to music after surgery in an intensive care unit showed reduced blood pressure and heart rate, less need for pain medication, and a 20 percent drop in two important stress hormones, epinephrine and interleukin-6 (IL-6). They also showed a surprising 50 percent jump in pituitary growth hormone, which can be associated with further reducing stress and jump-starting healing. These immediate and profound physiological changes with music are dramatic and can be easily used by anyone to heal.

With so much medical research backing the healing effects of music, Arts in Medicine programs are finding more and more ways to bring music into hospitals and care facilities to give patients this healing modality. Different music is introduced into different settings in hospitals, depending on the staff and patients. For instance, some hospitals bring musicians into public areas of hospitals, such as waiting rooms or, in some cases, into patients' rooms in hospital units. At Shands Arts in Medicine, there are weekly concerts, with string quartets, pianists, singers, and other musicians invited to play music in the open waiting areas. Musicians from the university and hospital community are also invited to play and participate. Medical students, artists, housekeeping staff, and nursing students all work together to create a concert series.

Another way to bring art into healthcare as a way of healing is by bringing music to the bedside, allowing patients and families to make requests from strolling musicians. In many hospitals, musicians wander the halls and go into patients' rooms to play guitar and sing, like minstrels from the Middle Ages. Music brings a powerful connection to the units in hospitals and creates beautiful experiences that are shared among patients' family and staff. Music is personal and individual, which means that each person is given the choice to select songs, albums, and artists to their personal liking. A guitar player can come into a patient's room where the patient is in pain and afraid. With one song, the space is altered and the patient is much more comfortable. This can be as powerful as pain medication, with no side effects.

With the super-portability of music today, music is now even used during procedures to relax and distract the patients and can be used before surgery, during lumbar punctures, or as a healing aid in other painful procedures. The patient just relaxes with earphones and listens to their iPod. If you (or someone you know) are going into a hospital or having a procedure, use a music player to play music to heal.

Healing music modalities that have become widespread in hospitals can become an important part of creating your own healing environment at home. Everything about music and healing is individual and personal. Different kinds of music evoke different kinds of memories and emotional states in each person. For healing, select music based on how it resonates with you. Feel the music in your own body. Does it change your emotions? Can you use it to deepen consciousness and produce calmness or serenity?

Any kind of music can be healing—jazz, classical, alternative, or rock. Music balances, produces harmony, relaxes, or stimulates. To heal, you can also choose music that energizes you and makes you feel powerful and strong. When you make your music selections, try to use them to create emotional states that work for you. For example, for medical procedures, people often choose deeply relaxing music, like soft bells or Mozart. For sleeping, they may choose lullaby-type songs or sounds of nature; for healing, they may choose hymns or psalms; for energy, maybe reggae or rock 'n' roll. Again, the music people choose is completely individual and personal.

You can make an intention to use music to evoke change in a moment, making it accessible to you at all times. You can use apps like Spotify to make albums for specific healing needs. Make the selections based on what makes you feel healthy, happy, and optimistic. Make choices based on what resonates naturally. When you use music, you need to be sensitive to how the music creates physical experiences. Say no to music if it makes you feel sick. Some music is hostile. Sounds come into our body as vibrations and integrate into our consciousness, so we need to choose music that creates wellness and promotes healing energy.

## *The Health Benefits of Listening to Music*

- Reduces pain
- Improves cognitive recovery and mood in patients who experience strokes
- Produces positive mood changes
- Decreases anxiety
- Decreases heart rate
- Decreases respiratory rate
- Decreases blood pressure
- Induces relaxation
- Promotes sense of power
- Lessens depression in patients with chronic nonmalignant pain
- Lessens sense of disability in patients with chronic nonmalignant pain
- Reduces nausea and vomiting in patients undergoing chemotherapy

## Delonzo's Story: Using Traditional African Music to Heal a Group

Delonzo Pope, one of Michael's students from his Art as a Healing course, said, "My drumming teacher always told us that when we play, we play to heal people, and I have seen and felt it for myself . . . playing music in a sacred space for a special purpose, using the gift of drumming to heal."

Delonzo is a tall, elegant African-American man with an unbelievable smile and wonderful healing energy. His energy is so positive and healing, you can't help but feel honored to be around him. When Delonzo became ill with pneumonia, he decided to change his career and his life. He was returning to school to study graphic design when he took Michael's class. He was a drummer, a martial arts instructor, and a healer.

When I heard that we could use any art medium we wanted to use for our final Medicine Art project for healing, I had a harder time than I thought I would trying to figure out what to do. Using an art form with the idea of healing is something I have always believed in. I've known for many years that art is therapeutic, and after the first week of the process I knew that this Caritas project, in any form, would be very moving to me.

My vision started out a little fuzzy, but after our second week together I decided that wanted to heal every one of my friends. I would use the ancient art of music to heal. I have a drum that is sacred to me: an African djembe. The djembe came from the Ivory Coast. It is made from one solid piece of wood from an old tree. When I hit it, it sang to me. My drumming teacher always told us that when we play, we play to heal people, and I have seen and felt it for myself. It is an African tradition to play drums and instruments to involve healing. They knew that music in this way could heal people, to involve the spirits of the ancestors, communicate, and give thanks to the Creator and the universe. This method of healing is thousands of years old and is still used today.

The art process that I would be using is the art of traditional polyrhythmic music that is four- to seven-hundred years old. I would heal my friends by playing a traditional song on my djembe and, if possible, get one or two other drummers to come help me. We call each other from time to time with hopes of getting together. I called some of my old classmates, told them my idea, and got two of my closest drumming friends to agree to help out. We agreed to no rehearsals and to just play the way our drumming teacher had taught us.

I came to the room next to the class where we would play and found myself in front of seven drummers. Two more of my friends had come to help, and they had brought additional drummers with them—all of them students of my drumming teacher. My heart sang out with thanks. We all hugged. We knew that this was going to be a special time. We then chose the most appropriate song we knew. We would do what our teacher had always talked about: play in a sacred space for a special purpose, using the gift of drumming to heal.

We entered the classroom and arranged ourselves into a semicircle in front of everyone, and I introduced the drummers and our intention. We were playing for the health of everyone involved. We left the lights off, with only the fading daylight to illuminate the room. We began playing a very old traditional song called "Positive." "Positive" is a very heavy and complex piece, with changes in speed, pitch, and rhythm that are designed to raise and fall with the rhythm of the nature world. Ocean, rain, storm, and the land are prime factors of the song as well. I observed the movements and gestures of my friends as well as the drummers while playing. The already electric room became much warmer, and the overall mood of the room became uplifted. Some people started moving to the beat; some started dancing. An intense energy could be felt in the room that during one of the most intense and energetic parts in the song, I had to play in increasing speed that transitions into a very heavy beat. It was then that my beloved djembe gave its last deep tonal healing beat and tore as I put my hand through the exhausted skin.

I felt sadness, release, and understanding all in the same instant. No other time could be more perfect to effect change and give up its energy to heal so many. The combined energy and love in that room touched me deeply. It hit me when we came close to the end of the song. I looked up and then realized that there were thirty healers in that room, a sacred space, playing ancient music and dancing freely. We did everything we had said we would do.

Delonzo was reviving the "boiling energy" concept that we brought up in week 2. Everyone involved in the dance and music, those participating and watching, were caught up in an ancient form of healing and helping each other connect to the source. This is the incredible power of music, where your thoughts, beliefs, and even your insides are rearranged and your body is healed.

**Lessons from Delonzo's Story**

- His goal was to heal the whole class. This was a courageous and large goal.
- He understood that music healed and strengthened his understanding with clear intent to make music to heal in a sacred space.
- He brought a group to help him and make it more powerful.
- The group made the music into ceremony.
- Music changed the environment.
- People danced and freed their own healing energy.
- He healed everyone and turned everyone into healers.

## Artist-Healer Profile: David Wilcox—Music as Shamanic Healing

"Music still stretches out before me like the headlights of a car into the night," said shaman musician David Wilcox. "It's way beyond where I am, but it shows where I'm going. I used to think that my goal was to catch up, but now I'm grateful that the music is always going to be way out in front to inspire me."

David's skills as a performer and storyteller are unmatched. He holds audiences rapt with nothing more than a single guitar, songs, and a fearless ability to mine the depths of human emotions of joy, sorrow and everything in between, and it's all tempered by a quick and wry wit. He asks people to tell their story. He says, "Tell me your thoughts, about an event, your feelings." Then he plays guitar, and like an oracle, he sings them a healing song for their soul. His intuitive abilities are uncanny. He taps into the part of himself that catches the slight wave of a feeling, which rushes over him and is translated into a profoundly healing song. He is shaman music-healer, a talented musician who has the capacity to create genuine, powerful, communicative songs that are beyond words. They are soul pieces. They have the intensity of what keeps us alive. It is about music transformed into shamanic healing in song.

I love hearing the perfect song at the perfect time, as if it's the soundtrack for what I'm living. Over the years, I've made up hundreds of songs that have worked like musical medicine to heal my heart and mind. But my favorite song to sing is the one that works for whom I'm singing it. So here are some songs organized by topic that might be just what the doctor ordered.

Following a series of gently probing questions aimed at tuning in to a participant's energy and divining their emotional truths, Wilcox performs what he calls "musical medicine," a personalized, poetically therapeutic song that speaks to the person's psyche in a powerful and profound way. His prescription poetry usually provokes smiles of recognition, if not flowing tears, that indicate that the harmonic remedy has resonated with the recipient on a deep level. Omega Institute cofounder Elizabeth Lesser, who cofacilitates annual workshops with David, simply calls him a shaman.

 Cathy Dewitt, a musician in residence at Shands Arts in Medicine, talks about the healing power of music and the joys of sharing it with patients. http://www.youtube.com/watch?v=mtiF9LAf1jg&list=PLMm-0ccB -CYpmKktLEws7WlrNyNg2QDnu&index=8

## Week 7 Praxis

We can become distracted by sounds of the television and recorded music. Return to the natural sounds of the earth and the rhythm of your own body.

Edie Hartshorne, a music healer, uses Tibetan bowls to heal. She told this story of listening and being healed by nature.

> I love no sound or the sound of fog. There is a quality of sound in fog that wraps you. I was in fog in a rainforest three years after my son died, and I felt an incredible intensity. I was very hot. I heard a voice, and I felt his presence all around me. In the fog I heard, "Haven't you noticed I have been here all the time? I have been with you always."

That was the moment, Edie said, when she was able to begin to heal. The focus of this guided imagery is to activate your experience of the sounds of nature.

### *Guided Imagery: Healing with Sounds of Nature*

Imagine yourself in a beautiful landscape. First, listen to the sound of the wind blowing through the leaves of trees. Now hear a hawk calling as it flies above you in the forest. Imagine sitting on the edge of a brook, listening to a waterfall as you watch a bird fly. Listen to the sound of the water bubbling over stones as it flows down the stream to the ocean. Hear the natural rhythm of the waves as they fluctuate in and out. Listen to the grasses moving, and feel the sound of the earth in your body. Listen to the sound of air moving, water flowing, earth moving, and fires sizzling. These elements surround us. Listen.

Continue to hear the sounds of the natural world as images come to you. Find a place in your imagination where you can simply listen. Experience the music of the earth's body. As you begin to hear these sounds, feel them going deeply into every cell of your own body. The vibration of these sounds enters you. Feel the sound as it resonates with the elements of your body. At this level of your experience, healing with sound takes place. The energy vibrates within your body and shifts into patterns that change and heal. Just by being inside the sound, you can soothe your body, re-pattern your body, and merge deeply within yourself. These sounds of nature are the songs of the earth. Listen to the earth singing to you. The earth's sounds are healing music.

As you listen to the rhythm of the earth's body, the sounds of the earth are moving into you and healing you. Listen to the subtle changes as the earth moves toward the sounds of a storm. The earth sings as thunder. The wind blows more strongly and then breathes softly into silence. The earth creates infinite musical sounds. She is always singing. The earth will heal you with her sound. Listen to the sound of the earth as it merges with the sounds of your own heartbeat and your own breath. Listen to the earth's song as your own song and let the earth sing to you. Listen; the song is the sound of her love for you.

In this moment, imagine yourself in the center of the earth's song. The sound of the earth's body resonates with you from before you were born until after you die. Her sound is infinite. Move into the sounds beneath your own breath and within the spaces between your heartbeat. This is the natural sound of your own body. When you listen to the sounds of your own body and the sounds of the earth, you create a perfect balance of becoming one with the sounds. Feel the sounds and rhythm flowing within your body, and feel the perfect harmony of these sounds as you listen. Let the sound surround you and hold you.

### Medicine Art: Make Music from Your Guided Imagery

Many people are intimidated by music and think they need to be accomplished musicians to play, especially in front of a group. In our classes, several students jump this barrier of their Inner Critic and for the first time play music, sing, or do both in front of everyone. This represents huge growth and a life-changing experience for them.

For this Medicine Art project, do something with music to heal. You can play music or listen to music with a clear intention to heal, sing, or play. Your ideas could come from the guided imagery or from anywhere. Pick an instrument—one you have played, a new one, or something really simple like a child's xylophone, drum, or harp. Play what comes to you, with the intention to heal. Or take those guitar or piano lessons you've been meaning to take, and learn a song that you can play by and from the heart. You can even just sing one note, chant, or hum. You can play a Tibetan bowl or a drum or meditate in silence. The following are some tips on how to incorporate music into your art-healing adventure to heal yourself, loved ones, friends and coworkers, or the world.

Find songs, chants, or drumming on YouTube, mp3, Soundcloud, Spotify, and so forth, and make an album that heals you. This is deeply personal; it is for you.

You can choose music for:

- Relaxation
- Excitement
- Dancing
- Freedom
- Deep healing
- Meditation
- Surgery preparation
- Use during a medical procedure
- Enlivening your workspace or home
- Background music or sound in large space, like a fountain
- White noise for a sleeping baby

The following are some ideas on other types of medicine music.

## *Drumming*

The drumbeat resonates deeply in the ancient human experience. The first sound we hear and connect to is a primordial one: our mother's heartbeat while we're in the womb. The Native American word for drum, *ad-we-gan*, means "heartbeat." Without drumming, ceremony would be impossible or even void. Drumming is a vehicle carrying participants deeper into their subconscious realms.

Drumming has been used throughout the history of humanity to create a trance state, a physiology that opens the mind and spirit. It is an excellent medium for transporting yourself into a deeper state of consciousness. The mind and body are able to move into the vibrational realms of sound and rhythm; the drum's rhythm balances brain waves to meditational states and shifts a person from frenetic, overactive brain waves to calmer, more self-regulated ones. Research, for example, has shown that drumming changes the brain-wave pattern from the high-frequency beta waves (the sometimes frenetic pattern of concentration and activity) to lower-frequency alpha and theta waves on the fringe of conscious and unconscious thought (the pattern of meditation, healing, trance, euphoria, and well-being). Delta waves, the lowest on the brain-wave spectrum, are the waves we produce during sleep. So music, by itself, changes our physiology from left-brain concentration to right-brain visionary states. Music, especially drumming, puts you in the state of mind to have visions, do guided imagery, and see spirit guides, spirit animals, ancestors, and so forth. That is why all Native American ceremonies are accompanied by drumming.

 Layne Redmond, a world renowned frame drummer, leads a healing ceremony. http://www.youtube.com/watch?v=wO4P25-vQiA&list=PLMm-0ccB -CYpmKktLEws7WlrNyNg2QDnu&index=9

## *Toning and Chanting*

Toning and chanting, like drumming, profoundly change body physiology. Simply toning one note from your inner center core relaxes you, drops blood pressure, and promotes healing. This is common in yoga. With chanting and toning, people experience altered states and natural highs caused by serotonin and dopamine release, which produces ecstatic feelings of bliss.

Gregorian chants and other Christian hymns have tones and rhythms that are particularly healing. Abbot Philip Lawrence, a scholar of chant who also leads the Monastery of Christ in the Desert, home to an American order of Benedictine monks, in Abiquiu, New Mexico, said, "The kind of singing that we do calms the spirit and helps us live in peace with our world and with one another. Chanting has some strange effect on the brain waves, according to various studies." The monks' goal is "to focus on the words rather than the challenge of voice production or sight reading. It is always our hope that our singing will bring others to peace, inner tranquility, and an appreciation of beauty. These values can help create a world in which peace and tranquility prevail."

Choral and religious music are also composed to put people in a physiology of prayer. Prayer, art, and healing all come from the same source, so when music alters consciousness to prayer, it changes our physiology, too. Choral and religious music from all cultures are often inspired by auditory visions and come from a higher consciousness to composers and musicians who meditate and pray.

Now these ancient modalities are more accessible to the mainstream and are being used more in hospitals and Arts in Medicine programs.

## Tibetan Bowls

Tibetan bowls, also called singing bowls, are ancient tools that have been used for centuries to create a particularly effective healing vibrational impact on the mind and body. Singing bowls are calibrated to create healing vibrational experiences and frequencies. Like the gentle ripples of a fallen leaf upon a pool of still water, the singing bowls can be used to shift and move energy that is felt vibrationally by an individual, a group, and the surrounding space or environment. A bowl's sound creates a pause, a transition, and a centering.

In the Tibetan tradition, these vibrational frequencies are attuned to the energy centers of chakras. Most commonly, they are

Root chakra—C
Sacral chakra—D
Solar plexus chakra—E
Heart chakra—F
Throat chakra—G
Third eye chakra—A
Crown chakra—B

The bowls actually sound as chords, with overtones that promote a shift of brain waves from the beta range to theta, where deep visions, spiritual visions, and dreams rise from the depths of our being. That is why many people use Tibetan bowls as a tool to do body work. Simply experiencing a singing bowl shifts the participant from a hyper-awake state of concentration and problem solving to a place of receiving visions to heal. This profound physiological shift is similar to advanced meditation or yoga practice.

A singing bowl healing is a process in which the person lies down on a blanket with seven Tibetan bowls surrounding their body. Bowls are placed above the head, below the feet, and around the body. The bowls are gently tapped to create powerful rhythmic sounds that facilitate deep relaxation. This opens the person's ability to go inside their body. The sound opens up the chakras, realigns the energy centers, promotes epiphanies, and facilitates powerful physiological healing states.

## Jean's Story: Healing with Music

Jean Watson is one of the leaders in caring science and art and healing in the world. Years ago a child hit her eye with a knife. To save her eye, she was put in bed in a way in which she was restrained and could not move her head at all. Her husband took wonderful care of her; he devoted himself to her and to saving her eye, but even after months of care, she lost it. Afterwards, her husband committed suicide and she entered a period of darkness in her life.

During this time she meditated, and one day, in her inner ear, she heard the most beautiful song she'd ever heard. Each day as she meditated, the song changed and grew stronger, more beautiful, and more healing. One day Jean realized they were not songs but psalms. They were music from a higher consciousness sent to her to heal.

As her practice grew, Jean became obsessed by the healing psalms she heard every day. She found a musician, and together they managed to sing, play, and record the songs that healed her and brought her from the darkness of an accident and loss to a very bright light of heavenly songs. She made a CD and shared her songs as healing for everyone. Jean was not a musician, but music healed her.

### Lessons from Jean's Story
- Going into the darkness begins the process of healing.
- Listening with the inner ear invites heavenly songs.
- Paying attention and honoring the process deepens it.
- Jean was not afraid that she was not a musician and did not listen to her Inner Critic.

- She invested work into finding a musician, recording, and making her CD.
- With music, Jean went from darkness to elsewhere, to making art as a turning point and transcendence.

## *Music and Community*

From antiquity to modernity, musicians have utilized rhythm, song, and acoustics as a way to both entertain and build community. When music that is familiar to a particular group is introduced, there is a dramatic response to music and song. You can witness and experience this in many ways—fans of a football team chanting and cheering for their team together, the audience at a rock concert singing along with the star, singing hymns with your church, or caroling during the holidays. Music is a wonderful vehicle to create an art-healing group. It is a physical phenomenon that creates vibrational resonance, holding people together in a way that is very powerful. When music is used as part of a healing ceremony, it unites people and their consciousness. The healing force can be shared by the community or done for the sake of another person or for a specific cause.

This week, if you have an art-healing group, see who is a musician. If you're solo, play music for yourself. Pick an instrument and play. Sing along with music you are listening to. Write your own songs and play them on anything. Sing songs you know—old folk songs, rock songs, Native American healing songs, and so forth. For this practice, imagine that Delonzo is with you, drumming in the background, laughing, and telling you how wonderful you are. He is like a classmate of yours in the universal class of art and healing.

### Artist-Healer Profile: Therese Schroeder-Sheker—Music at the End of Life

Another important and beautiful use of music is facilitating peaceful transitions at the end of life. There is an emerging field of musicians committed to creating healing environments that grant the experience of peace and release from the body's suffering.

Therese Schroeder-Sheker was one of the first artists to use a harp at end of life. She was dean of the School of Music-Thanatology in Missoula, Montana, and helped create the field of music-thanatology, where musicians play for those who are dying.

Music-thanatology has been shown to reduce physical and emotional pain, create a supportive environment, and help people have a conscious death process. This is an incredible resource that is under-recognized. Music invites the listener to transience into the lightness of vibrational embodiment. Many hospices and hospitals now have music-at-end-of-life programs.

*Checklist: Healing with Music*

**Step One: Starting on the Path**

- Find a time each day and listen to music consistently.
- Pick music you love that resonates with you.
- Turn your phone off.
- Close your eyes and listen.
- Let music take you elsewhere.
- Breathe with the music.
- Get in touch with each sound.
- Return to the pleasure of music.
- Find a place to sing, tone, or chant.
- Experience the sounds of nature.

**Step Two: The Creative Journey to Heal**

- Make music an intentional part of healing activities.
- Play music to relax.
- Listen to music that is healing.
- Bring music to any stressful event by making your own music library.
- Say no to hostile or jarring sounds.
- Go to sound with intention to balance.
- Become one with the sound.
- Feel the rhythm in your body.
- Hum or chant.
- Sing or repeat words to a rhythm.
- Sing in the shower.
- Tone in the shower.
- Try playing an instrument like a child does, with joy and without judgment.
- Learn to play a new instrument.
- Walk along a stream or brook and listen.
- Find the music of the ocean, brook, or waterfall and listen.
- Listen to the wind and fog.

- Listen to birds.
- Feel the harmony of sound surrounding you.

## Step Three: Deepening

- Feel the power rise within you.
- Allow the vibrational shifts in your body to move through you.
- Repeat affirmations such as "I am one with my song" to music.
- Sing lullabies to yourself or a loved one.
- Listen to the music of your enemy.
- Invite friends to serenade you with music.
- Ask a friend to play the guitar and sing to you.
- Make your own instrument with found objects.
- Use repetitive sound rhythms as an inner chant.

## Step Four: Transcendence

- Imagine your spirit soaring as song.
- Sing to your bones.
- Sing from your heart.
- Evoke your God with music and song.
- Learn sacred chants.
- Listen to silence.
- Put yourself in the center of a healing circle of music.
- Make a drumming circle for healing.
- Listen to the earth's body sing to you.
- Turn up the volume of nature's healing music.
- Create a community of music makers.
- Form singing circles.
- Let the music carry you to a Higher Power.

## Summary of Week 7

- Do the guided imagery for the sounds of nature.
- Make a music album for you to use to heal.
- Play an instrument as complicated as a piano or as simple as a child's xylophone.
- Chant, tone, or use a Tibetan bowl to change your physiology to heal.
- Do guided imagery while you listen to a drumming CD or Tibetan bowl CD.
- Write music, compose music, and sing or play; then ask someone do it for you.

# WEEK 8

# HEALING WITH DANCE AND MOVEMENT

*Divine dancer, emerge from within. Open our bodies to experience the freedom of being alive. Move, flow, and touch the inner grace and integrity of the movement of life itself. May the divine dancer move and let the body be the story, myth, and beauty.*

In ancient times, the movement of dance was used for prayer and healing. It was used to build inner fire, increase energy, and release energy, like the boiling energy of the Bushmen and the dances of other indigenous cultures. Similarly, in tai chi and yoga our relationship with the environment produces balance. Our bodies become a meditation and an embodiment. Movement produces a fusion of mind, body, and spirit.

With dance and movement, you can experience grace, beauty, and fun. It's about inviting openness, naturalness, and flow. Movement creates warmth, frees energy, and changes physiology. It stimulates your whole body. Dance heals by releasing tensions so we can connect to deep ancient patterns. The patterns are healing; when you embody them, your body heals.

It is important to move in your body because movement is physical and it is life. It allows your spirit to completely permeate every cell and part of your body, from head to fingers, from your core to your legs and toes. Movement and dance is as natural as breathing. When we dance to heal ourselves, others, our community, or the earth, we are releasing the spirit by unwinding the body. Inside your body there is a free spirit, a natural dancer. Connect to this part of you with freedom. It is your Inner Healer stirring.

Movement is a basic, essential part of life. When you get out of bed and move through space and time, you can feel yourself naturally dancing in your everyday life. Fluidity in moving through our environment is part of walking or running. As creatures, we have evolved to these natural movements that free energy. Instead of rushing, you have an opportunity to shift into an embodiment of movement, deepening your ability and awareness to move from your core.

When you create a deliberate, conscious movement, you interface with the environment and harness the energy around. You can flow and move with rhythm in the surrounding environment. The dance of life is as natural to us as the action of a butterfly moving from flower to flower or a lion chasing prey. Connect to the natural movements in your body.

With every movement, you embody your own inner creative fire. Imagine yourself as a dancer. The dancer within you is beautiful, liberated, and free. In everyday moments, you can use the grace of the dance with the rhythm and motion of your body. This creates a subtle shift in your perspective. As you move from the core centeredness of your own being, you can harness the connection with intention and grace. The dancer within you is the seducer and seductress, the artist who creates the healing spiral.

## Bear Dancing

Michael bear dances three times a year with Native Americans to heal people and communities. Bear dancers wear a bearskin and dance with bear movements, growling and scratching. Then the ancient healing power of the bear spirit arrives.

The Native Americans Michael dances with believe that the dancer carries the healing bear spirit. The bear spirit is the real healer. Dancers carry the bear, and the human disappears during the dance. The bear helps the people release the illness and heal.

Using the bearskin, Michael has also worked with women with breast cancer. When he put the bearskin on them and invited them to dance the bear, they told him that the fear left them. Their courage came because there was not room for both cancer and the bear when they danced as bear.

Michael leads a bear dance with a woman to heal.
http://www.youtube.com/watch?v=jHRVe_iu6LM&list=PLMm-0ccB
-CYpmKktLEws7WlrNyNg2QDnu&index=1

This kind of art is healing because it's transformational. When the artist-healer, priestess, or shaman transforms into the spirit animal, the animal spirit takes over the healer and the healing process. This is the secret to healing through animal transformations. The dancer does not do the healing; it's done by the animal spirit and the person who is ill. Native American Stanford-trained physician and author Lewis Mehl-Mardrona eloquently wrote in his book *Coyote Medicine*, "Only the Creator and the spirits, or the patient, can really take credit for a healing." He explained that the shaman is only with them. Native Americans won't say they are shaman or that they do the healing; we need to be humble or the spirits leave us. Lewis Mehl-Madrona continued, "One Apache I revered told me, 'The patient does 70 percent of the work to get well, the Creator does 20 percent, and I do 10, which is barely worth mentioning.' Most of what the patient does to get well, he told me, is make the firm decision to *be* well."[2]

The healing in the ancient indigenous spirit animal dance is about the person and spirit animal, not healers, gurus, or therapists. This is a very different view of healing from allopathic medicine's drugs and surgery.

Seeing through the eyes of a spirit animal, wearing the skin of an animal, being the spirit animal in your imagination, turning into the animal in guided imagery, and dancing the animal fuses modern and ancient technology, combining animal transformation and the basic roots of spiritual healing and art and healing.

 Inna Dagman, a student in Michael's class at San Francisco State University and a dance healer, talks about discovering her love and passion for dance through the Art as a Healing Force program, and how the expression of movement is incredibly healing.
http://www.youtube.com/watch?v=E3BTILj9Nyc&list=PLMm-0ccB -CYpmKktLEws7WlrNyNg2QDnu&index=8

## Maria's Story: Tears in Heaven

*I almost subconsciously used music for myself as a healing agent,*
*and lo and behold, it worked . . . I have gotten a great deal of happiness*
*and a great deal of healing from music.*

—Eric Clapton, musician

---

2. Lewis Mehl-Madrona, *Coyote Medicine: Lessons from Native American Healing* (New York: Fireside, 1997), 122.

Dancing freely and just moving can become a doorway to deep healing. Maria, a student at University of Florida, did not know what to do for her project but knew she loved to dance. One day she just went outside and began to move. She told us,

I looked out my window. Beautiful flowers were blooming outside, and the sun was out. It was so beautiful that I decided to dance free, like the flowers. I went outside and put on my favorite music. By this time, the sun was setting; I could see shadows in the beautiful oak trees all around me. It was so beautiful. I started to dance, moving to the feeling, seeing how far my body could move.

Then I imagined myself as a true dancer. The next song came on my music player. It was Eric Clapton's "Tears in Heaven." Suddenly I was moving. I had a memory of the child I had lost. The song and movement triggered a memory. *Who would I recognize in heaven?* I thought as I danced. I knew that Eric Clapton has written this song after he'd lost a child, and what came up for me was my memory of losing my child. I could feel and recognize this child as I danced. As I danced, I had an image of a little boy. I saw him, and I danced to him.

Sadness came up. Suddenly in my dance body, I took emotions. I danced in sorrow, a deeper dance. Then I saw my living children. I saw the child I had lost between my living children. I saw all of them. Then as I continued dancing, the other children faded, and I stayed and danced with the child I had lost. I danced with him at the age he would have been; in that moment, he would have been twenty-one years old. I danced a dance of forgiveness, a dance with loss and grief. Then the child slipped into the body of my youngest son. In my imagination, I could now love this lost child by loving my youngest child.

The dance was profound and healing. In my memory, I never saw this child I had lost, and I never spoke to him. Now in the dance I was suddenly dancing with him. It was a beautiful experience.

## Revisiting Inna: Healing My Mother and Myself with Dance

Inna told us about how she healed her mother with dance.

For my final Medicine Art project, I was supposed to engage in healing art of any type and present it to someone. I immediately knew that I wanted to do something for my mom, to help her with her severe depression. My parents had recently separated. They had been married forever, with three children, a house, a full life. We had moved many times and been through a lot, but this was something more. I was old enough to have my own life, but my mother was devastated and depressed. Our family was torn apart—finished, really—and she was alone. She wasn't eating or sleeping much. Anytime I saw her, she looked like the life in her had died. My beautiful mother, who had lovingly raised three daughters, was in the lowest of places, and it was breaking my heart. My whole family, even my dad, was extremely worried. We all carried this huge pain with us during that time. So as soon as the words "healing project" were spoken, I knew I was going to help her somehow.

I had no idea that this project would become a portal for my own personal transformation and a reunification with my inner artist-healer core. The day of my project presentation, I invited my mom to come with me.

No one had ever brought a family member to our class. It was courageous, creative, and full of clear, powerful intent. Inna sat her mother on the floor on a cushion. I can only imagine how her mother felt, sitting in the center of a circle with a class of people she did not know around her. She looked apprehensive but strangely calm.

Inna put on a piece of music and slowly started to dance around her mother. As she danced, Inna seemed to change; she became a healing spirit, an angel. Her body movements flowed, dipped, and rose like a bird or a healing goddess. She was almost invisible. We were all entranced. And then, almost magically, the movements became pure love. It was not a woman and a dancer; it was a dyad of love that came from above and flowed through the dance to Inna's mother.

Her mother lit up, becoming larger and stronger, and so did we. I don't remember if Inna actually kissed and hugged her mother or told her she loved her; her love was so huge, it was portrayed in the dance. Inna's dance encompassed her mother, covered her like a blanket of love, and came out of space and time from a sacred place of perfect beauty. Everyone in the room was healed by this love.

This is how Inna told this part of the story:

For my presentation, I chose a beautiful song and danced a healing dance for my mother. I had never before danced in front of strangers without rehearsing, and with such emotion and sacredness. The movements seemed to flow out of a deep place within me—a place of no judgment, complete acceptance and love, and healing energy. As I danced, something shifted in me and in the whole room. I knew that something magical was happening—and it wasn't my ego. It was a healing presence, a doorway that opened. My mother's intense pain was being safely held by the dance, healing energy, and unconditional love. What was happening was much larger than my personality or my dance ability. It was coming from elsewhere, from a pure place of healing, and I was channeling that energy in my movements. I had no idea what happened. But I knew that it was magical, and that it happened because my intention to heal and a safe and loving space were present. To this day, both my mom and I remember this day as one of the most moving experiences in our lives.

The day I danced a healing dance for my mom, something woke up inside me. Although I didn't know it at the time, I glimpsed my purpose and my future. However, I still had some obstacles to face before returning to the path toward healing dance. After I graduated, my life became consumed by work, and I was dancing very little. Soon I started doctoral studies in psychology, and at that point I wasn't dancing at all. I became disillusioned, depressed, and physically ill. I wasn't finding fulfillment in my studies, and I lost touch with my core and my healing abilities. One day, with the help of a wise friend, I reached a turning point and decided to quit my studies. This began the process of healing my life and reconnecting with my core and spirit. I didn't know yet where I was heading, but I did know that there are two things I must do right away: reconnect with art and healing and start dancing.

With this process, I experienced transformation, inspiration, and a healing creativity. It was the first time I have encountered qualities of sacredness, complete acceptance, lack of judgment, and healing love. Those elements moved me deeply and invited me to connect with my inner core.

Inna has made dance-healing her life work. She is now interning with Jill Sonke, the dancer-in-residence at University of Florida, and is Mary's teaching assistant in her course Spirituality and Creativity in Healthcare at the University of Florida. She is doing dance with Parkinson's patients, the elderly, and people in hospitals to free the dancer-healer within.

Inna continued,

The Art as a Healing Force process has opened up a well inside me. I didn't use to think of myself as a creative person, but I found out that there was an enormous spring of creative life inside of me, and as soon as the invitation came, it started to flow. I know that each of us has this beautiful spring deep inside. It sits there quietly, waiting to be acknowledged. And maybe the longer it is ignored, the harder it is to reconnect to it. But I have seen that spring open up in all the people who took Michael's class, and I see it now that I am assisting in Mary's class. People might say that they are not creative, but as the weeks go by, something shifts, and all this beautiful creativity begins to flow from a place that was previously unacknowledged. That sacred spring opens up every time there is an invitation to create with the intent to heal, to hear the voice of one's spirit.

I have made this work and process my life.

After her internship with the Arts in Medicine program at the University of Florida, Inna planned to return home to California and help bring this healing process to hospitals and clinics, where it is not part of the structure yet. She dances every day and plans on developing healing dance workshops to help people get back into their bodies and connect with the sacred dancer within them. "The Art as a Healing Force process," she said, "has healed and completely changed my life."

**Lessons from Inna's Project**
- Sometimes when you are art and healing in action, you know that is who you are when you start the twelve-week process.
- Healing dance comes from a place deep within us, full of emotion and love.
- It helps your creativity to have a sacred place of nonjudgment.

**Artist-Healer Profile: Anna Halprin—Animal Transformations and Dance**

Anna Halprin, director of the Tamalpa Institute in Marin County, California, is the grandmother of healing dance. She has taught many people to use dance to heal, and she leads an annual dance for peace in the mountains outside San Francisco.

One beautiful day we sat on her deck in a forest of tall redwood trees. She invited a cancer patient she was working with to dance as his power animal. He was a young man, thin and weak-looking. He sat in the sun and did a guided imagery. He saw a turtle as his spirit animal. He got down on all fours of the deck and moved slowly, raising each foot and arm and putting each down slowly. He became a turtle in front of our eyes. We could see his shell and see him carry its weight. He moved around the deck in a slow circle, looking stronger and stronger as he danced with his heavy shell.

Afterwards, he told us that this dance gave him great strength. It gave him the protection and grounding he needed to face his difficult treatment ahead. When a person dances the movements of the spirit animal, the body memories of being that animal are freed from the spiritual DNA and its power emerges. For instance, when a person dances bear, the person becomes strong, courageous, and powerful. When a person like this young man dances turtle, they have protection.

## Week 8 Praxis

Now we are going to do a guided imagery to release and illuminate your dancer within.

### *Guided Imagery: Seeing Yourself as a Dancer*

As you relax, allow your body to soften. Just pause, releasing any tension and any preoccupation with anything you need to do or somewhere you need to go. In this moment, simply sit on your chair or lie on the ground and feel your experience of being in your body. Now we will do a body scan, starting with your toes. In your mind's eye, feel the connection with your toes and the soles of your feet. Feel the connection to the earth; feel the journey you have taken with your feet, where they have taken you. Allow yourself to be connected to each of your feet. As you imagine yourself grounded with your feet on the earth, imagine there are spirals going up your calves. Feel the energy go up each calf, up your knees, up your thighs. Feel the connection of your feet, knees, and thighs. You are balanced.

Now imagine in your mind's eye your pelvis and the trunk of your body. Feel the strength of your body as you lie or sit. Become aware of your spine, from your coccyx to your neck. Feel the spiral energy ascending. Now imagine the energy moving through your trunk and down your arms, elbows, and forearms, until you feel the energy in each finger. If you feel the desire to move, let your body do this. Move fluidly if that feels comfortable to you.

Now imagine the energy in your neck going up through your face, head, lips, nose, and eyes, up to the top of your head. For a moment, connect to the still point in your body and in your mind's eye, see the energy spiraling up your limbs and trunk. You sense inner movement beginning to stir. Breathe into your body, feeling the embodiment of all aspects of your body: your bones, muscles, nerve endings, skin—your entire form and shape.

In this moment, your body is the starting point. Allow yourself to remain grounded and connected to the earth. Feel your body standing. Using your mind's eye, not your actual body, allow your body to begin to move ever so softly and slowly. In the beginning, feel your fingers begin to move. Allow them to open and close in your mind's eye, and explore the delicacy of each movement. Now imagine your arms gently moving through space, making a variety of movements around your head. Let them move across your body to form a *T* shape; then move down to your thighs. Now, staying in your mind's eye, begin moving your shoulders and neck. Explore the sensation of moving in your body with your mind's eye.

Now gently move your actual body—your physical form. Slowly experience the exploration of a movement. As you do this, experiment with moving your body with your eyes closed. Move your neck side to side, your head backwards and forwards. Begin to experience this gentle natural flow of your body, bending to the front, to each side. Move slowly enough to feel the sensual connection and naturalness of each movement. Move as slowly as possible. Allow your body to move naturally in the way that feels the most comfortable and fluid. Just move as your body wants to move. Keep your eyes closed, exploring the different movements of your body. As you are moving, imagine a central point inside your body that you are dancing around—an inner core. Explore the movement around this point. It is the sun that you rotate around. Give yourself permission to dance around the beautiful sun in the center of your body. As you begin to move, you may feel tightness or discomfort. Focus on this area with a gentle movement. Play, experiment, and allow your movements to vibrate around the part of you that is calling you. Invite this part of yourself to begin to move and find its own rhythm. Now simply allow yourself to move. Open yourself to the possibility of different movements.

As you move, imagine yourself as a dancer with total freedom of movement. Allow your body to follow the images in your mind as much as you can. In your mind's eye, extend your movement beyond its limitation. Allow new possibilities and see yourself as a dancer, free and liberated. Allow your body to gently follow your imagery the best it can. As the dancer within comes out, allow it to move without fear. Dance with your body as the dancer in your mind's eye.

Now come to your place of stillness, inviting that dancer to become part of who you are. Invite the inner dancer to merge with your body and soul. Breathe this dancer into your body. Imagine the dancer illuminated within your body.

In guided imagery space, your feet are grounded. There is a spiral energy moving around your central axis. You move in alignment around the axis and are balanced. You move with the energy from the earth harnessed in your body. It energizes you deeply. You are connected and deeply expanded. You use your body to fluidly harness the energy coming through you; you use the energy intentionally. You are connected to the earth and moving from centeredness and alignment. We are all capable of being in balance with the sun inside our chest, and we are rotating around it like the earth. Connect and harness these energies. Come from balance and grounding.

Relax. Take several deep breaths. Let your breathing slow. Allow your abdomen to rise when you breathe in and fall when you breathe out. See yourself as a beautiful healing dancer. See yourself dancing around someone who is ill. See your movements healing them. See healing energy come out of your hands, feet, and heart. See the healing light around you as you dance.

### *Medicine Art: Embodiment with Dance*

First we will use our breath to warm up and get ready. To breathe in, feel your breath fill your entire chest and abdomen. Now allow your breath to fill your fingers, legs, and toes. Using dance is like unraveling your body to free your spirit. Your body is moving as you unwind yourself so your spirit can be free and dance.

Awaken your inner dancer, choose your favorite music, and begin to dance. In the beginning, you may be hesitant to dance. Recognize that your body yearns for movement to experience its own lightness of being and create inner healing. Create space in your own home, living room, or porch and allow yourself to enter this space. Imagine yourself moving in this space. Allow yourself to experience the expressive nature of your body. In the beginning it may feel awkward or alien. This is normal; it's okay. Allow yourself to move despite any fears about the way it looks or feelings of awkwardness in your body. You are a natural dancer, even if you can't imagine it.

Imagine in your mind's eye freedom and spontaneity without limitations. Close your eyes and feel what it's like to stand still with your eyes closed. Put your hands over your head and stretch out your body, gently and slowly. Feel the luxury and sensuality of your body moving through space. Feel your natural movements of grace, of being totally embodied. Open your eyes. As you open them, gently let yourself explore motion with your hands, your entire arms, your waist, and both sides, and move your legs. Explore the full range of motion in your body. Feel the incredible pleasure and delight in movement.

Dance is simply moving in a sequential form of gestures using your hands, arms, legs, and gestures of opening, closing, standing, bending, moving downward, and moving upward. Dancing means moving your limbs and exploring possible ranges of motion. You can begin with exercise techniques and practice with rhythm, integrating music and rhythm. Invite yourself to feel the freedom of your own natural way of moving. Your initial strategy is to bring dance into your own home environment, create a time to dance, and make it a part of your life. Allow your dancing to explore your personal environment. Dance to your favorite music. Dance because no one is watching. Challenge yourself to be playful. Allow your body to express emotions through dance. Imagine a situation and dance it out. Allow yourself to move, your dance unfolding unconsciously.

Don't worry about understanding what is evolving; dance is a discovery. If a dance is intense or difficult, move into those feelings and express them in your body. You don't need to define or understand what emerges and becomes transformed. The focus of the dance is to re-create feelings from an event or make it up. As you become the dancer, let the dancer move you.

To begin with, allow yourself to dance for twenty to thirty minutes each day. Allow your dance to take form. After each dance, appreciate your body and your ability to move to the extent you can. Appreciate your dance as a healing experience.

Dancing is deeply personal. Its purpose is to let you experience the beauty of your body. Let the dance take you inside yourself to a spacious and deeper reality. Allow the dance to move you into memories, forms, and feelings, giving your inner dancer permission to move more deeply into what your body remembers.

Dance creates your experience of wholeness. We invite you to dance to feel deeply connected to your own life. In the beginning you may feel a separateness. Move into that space, allowing your body to merge with the dancer. Do not condemn any gesture you do; continue with openness. In the beginning, move very slowly, following your feelings. Your emotional body will lead your physical body in new ways of moving. In each movement, pay attention to the moment. It may be helpful to work with imagery. Explore imagery as it evolves into a feeling state. Your body has a rhythm connecting it to the core of your own aliveness—your heartbeat, breath, and natural, exquisitely orchestrated order.

Begin to explore your awareness of your own rhythm. It could be your own awareness of feelings that move into expression. Explore the expansion of movement inviting the expression of freedom. Allow yourself the freedom to experience the unknown again and again. It may be easier to work with music that resonates with your own rhythm. The goal is to use rhythmic art to fully express your wholeness. Experience ecstasy and sadness. Your dance embodies your own harmony, melody, and rhythm; your body, mind, and spirit are expressed as one. In this alignment, bliss and healing take place.

The next three basic dances are exercises we do with our art-healing groups. Two are done with partners. Dance is often performed with another person; and dancing someone's story for them can be deeply healing for both people. So if you want to do these exercises, find a partner to work with. It can be a friend, your life partner, or someone you are working with the Art as a Healing Force process. You can dance the third dance by yourself if you don't have a partner to work with.

### First Medicine Art Dance: Dance a Tree, Dance Your Spirit Animal

Many dancer-healers use this exercise as the first exercise for dance. You can do it solo. It is very simple. In your mind's eye, see a tree—a mystical tree, an ancient sacred tree. Now be this tree. Stand with your roots in the ground, your limbs aloft, and your leaves blowing in the gentle breeze. Move as the tree moves. Feel the tree and move like you feel. This exercise is easy and really fun. Keep going, dancing your tree.

Now imagine an animal. If you have a spirit animal, call it to you. Otherwise, dance any animal that comes to mind, without censorship. Invite the animal to come to you and into your body. Put on fur, claws, a beak, or whatever your animal has. Dance your animal. Let your animal dance you. Move like your animal. Let your animal move you. Make animal sounds. Move, stand, fly, swim, and climb. Let the animal come into your body and be the animal. See out of its eyes and move as it would.

You can do this in a big space or in a small space. You can do this as a ceremony to heal another person. When you do this simple exercise, you are in good company. Many of the best dancer-healers have patients dance their power animal to heal. Your spiritual DNA remembers the animal movements and takes on the attitudes of the animal. So if you dance bear, you have courage, strength, and power. Native Americans believe that when you carry an animal, you take on its powers and its spirit comes to heal. So dance your animal now.

### *Second Medicine Art Dance: Being Led in a Dance with Eyes Closed*

This exercise needs to be done with a partner. Take turns with a partner leading each other to move, walk, or dance. Some people find it easier to be led while others prefer to lead. Your first exercise is to be led for five minutes. Close your eyes while your partner leads. This exercise is done with no music. Allow your partner to simply move you so you can experience being led. Your partner honors your limitations and creates a flow to help you explore your repertoire of movements. You and your partner are connected. As you are being led, practice surrender, trust, and faith that you are safe. Focus inside your body, gently moving through space as you are led around. Keep your eyes closed; allow yourself to have fun and be light. You may feel awkward or have a sense that the exercise is too long, but this is part of the experience. Move through your own resistance and stay in your body. Focus inward. Feel your hands and arms; feel and move through space and time. Let go of control.

Now switch roles. You are now the leader. Lead the movements of your partner and take them on a dance, leading them. Explore deeply, moving up and down, stretching limbs out, expanding the movements, and warming up. You can hold your partner by the hands and lead them gently and carefully in a dance. Hold hands as you move and create a dance with flow and rhythm. Use your own internal rhythm in connection with your partner's. This is beautiful and fun, a deep and powerful exercise. With this exercise, you learn about trust, connections, surrender, leading, caring, and touch. You cultivate trust, faith, and a sense of being taken care of. You create deep, magical relationships beyond words that prepare you for the next exercise.

### *Third Medicine Art Dance: Tell a Story of an Illness, Listen,*
### *and Dance It as a Dancer-Healer*

This exercise can be done with your partner from the previous exercise, or you can work solo. For this powerful exercise, you will share a story of a lived experience of an illness or something you want to heal. Recall a memory as it was experienced in your body.

What were you thinking? What happened, and how did you feel? Tell your story from your physical memory, not just your mind. It does not have to be a serious illness or very personal story if you are not comfortable with that. It can be something very simple.

If you are doing this exercise with a partner, let the other person listen without speaking as you share your story for three minutes. Then pause, breathing in and out. Center yourself and rest in silence, sit, and hold your story.

Now the listener will dance your story as a healing dance. The listener becomes the dancer and dances your story. For three minutes, the dancer creates whatever movement feels real to them as a dancer-healer. Your story is shared and reflected back to you as a healing dance. Allow the story to have a beginning, a middle, and an end. When it is done, the dancer sits down.

Now switch roles. Your partner tells their story of an illness experience or what they want healed. They tell you what they lived and what actually happened. You simply listen quietly, holding their story. Now you will dance their story back to your partner.

You can do this exercise alone, dancing your own story for yourself. You can dance a story of someone else, a family member, someone you are working with, or an absent person. This exercise is your experience to dance a story as a dancer-healer. The experience is different; when you dance someone else's story, you heal another person, and when you dance your own story, you heal yourself. Both ways you are a dancer-healer, using the experience of dance to heal.

This exercise is powerful. By moving your body, listening, and using your body, you reflect the story back as healer, healing with dance. The experience is very powerful and very real and allows you to move though resistance that comes up when you use your body more fully. It allows you to feel what it is like to be a dancer-healer. Make sure to share with your partner your experience and what your dances meant to each other.

### *Medicine Art: Write These Experiences in Your Journal.*

Write about what it felt like to dance an animal; what if felt like to be led with your eyes closed; and what it felt like to be a dancer-healer and to dance someone's story to heal them.

## *Checklist: Healing with Dance*

**Step One: Starting on the Path**
- Find a space to be your dance floor where your movement can be free.

- Stretch and warm up daily.
- Connect with the energy inside your body.
- Allow your body to move spontaneously; follow the movements.
- Select music you love or want to move to.
- Let the rhythm of life be your music.
- Transform your ordinary movements into a sacred dance.
- Walk through your life with the grace of a dancer.
- Start to dance, exploring pure movement.
- Allow the divine dancer to move within you.

## Step Two: The Journey of the Creative Dancer to Heal

- See each movement as a deliberate, conscious act.
- Make an intention to move in beauty and grace.
- Embody emotions as movements.
- Use your breath to create an ebb and flow.
- Use scarves to move air in flowing movements or to simulate water.
- Access your inner self through dance.
- Go to the place where emotion merges with movement.
- Allow sounds to emerge as you dance, if that is natural.
- Be nonjudgmental and let go of criticism or expectation.
- Merge with the life force.
- Dance to music of your enemy.
- Dance in community with friends and foes.

## Step Three: Deepening Your Dance Process

- Dance within the motions of your day.
- Draw images and then dance them.
- Dance symbols.
- Dance an animal.
- Dance a tree or rock.
- Dance an image or a feeling.
- Move to define space.
- Go deep inside your body.

- If you dance with others, make a lot of contact; don't be afraid of appropriate touching.
- Dance someone's story of an illness to heal them.
- Use imagery in your dance.
- Dance to connect with your soul.

**Step Four: Dance as Transcendence**
- Visualize your spirit and body becoming one.
- Feel yourself as a dance of pure light.
- Allow yourself to fall deeply into the center of a dancing spiral.
- Allow yourself to dance through life as you move.
- Receive the energy of the earth.
- Connect with the dancer in the stars.
- Honor the mystery of the dance.
- Dance as one in whirling circles with people in conflict.
- Create a sacred circle of witnesses to your dance.

# Summary for Week 8

- Do the guided imagery to see yourself as a dancer.
- Dance a spirit animal or tree.
- Dance with another person with your eyes closed.
- Dance a story of your own illness or another person's illness to heal.

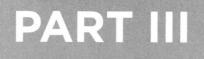

# PART III

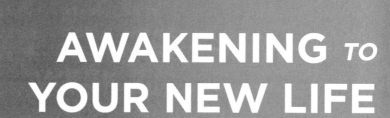

# AWAKENING *TO* YOUR NEW LIFE

# Awakening to Your New Life

This part of our book is about finding your essence and working with deep issues that may need to be healed. The twelve-week process is effective for all kinds of mental, emotional, and physical healing, but finding meaning in life, embracing your sexuality, and coming to terms with mortality are three very common themes in our classes, as well as in final Medicine Art projects. Addressing these issues is essential to healing the whole person, so we will take a week to work with each. In the course of part 3, you'll learn new ceremonies that combine media together for intentional healing. This will make the art and healing even more powerful. In our last week, we conclude our time together with the completion of your final Medicine Art project and a graduation ceremony.

# WEEK 9

# FINDING YOUR ESSENCE

*Our essence is found; it is only a matter of seeing it there before us
and knowing its truth—for it is time to share.*

One of the goals of the art-healing process we've been guiding you through is to help you find your essence, your authentic self, and your gifts. It is our hope that this creative process has enlightened your experience of yourself. This week we will use the wisdom, insight, and your inner witness to develop a deeper consciousness of who you truly are and why you are here. Each of us is born with a gift. The gifts are often lost under our life stories; they are hidden by painful things that happened to us as children and adults. Art and healing are about finding your own special gift and living them as your new life.

In this chapter, we share a story about Vijali Hamilton, an incredible artist-healer, who used art as way of healing to make peace. Vijali's story is the inspiring tale of one woman who decided to awaken in her life and find her essence, which led her to completely redirect her life and start using art to heal the world. It is a story of vision, total commitment and honesty, and giving up everything to become an artist-healer for peace on earth. We hope it inspires you to search for your own life's meaning and purpose as we continue to make Medicine Art. Finding and embracing your essence also factor heavily into your final project.

## Vijali's Story: World Wheel

Vijali was a successful artist selling beautiful carved stone sculptures in galleries in Los Angeles, California. She was married and had a secure comfortable life but felt unfulfilled and empty. Something irresistible was calling her to a new life. So she decided to leave her life behind, and she became a hermit, living completely alone in a trailer in the mountains outside Malibu, California, in a place called Boney Mountain. Her small trailer had no water or electricity. She stayed there in meditation for five years. In her meditation during the time she spent alone, she had a vision. She told us this story.

I returned from a trip to find myself in a struggle to live in simplicity—a simplicity I had difficulty finding in Santa Monica with my husband. My days were filled with a longing for the mountains. Running through my mind like a mantra were the words, "Where is our sacred mountain?" I needed to integrate two worlds—the world of nature that so easily fostered understanding of our connection with all life and the world created by society, government, schools, advertisements, television, parents, and all forces that push us to feel we are separate from nature, from our natural selves. Those forces tell us we need new clothes and cars and thin, beautiful bodies to be happy. I told my husband, "I feel an urgency to honor the sacredness of the Santa Monica Mountains by living with the rhythms of nature and my own unfolding nature." The next month, I moved into the trailer on Boney Mountain, in a place bordering the National Forest. I had the feeling that I had found my sacred space in the backyard of Los Angeles. Here was where I intended to live without the compromise of leading a double life.

During my retreat on Boney Mountain, I had a vivid dream one night that steered the course of my life back into the world. In this dream, I saw myself carving giant sculptures out of living rock, creating sacred sites in countries I had never visited before. The people in these communities spoke languages I had never heard. At the end of my stay in each country, we performed a ceremony of transformation with music, dance, and ritual for our lives, their community, and the world. I went from country to country around the globe to create a giant circle of peace. The conviction of my dream was that within this circle there was so much upheaval and bloodshed—in the Middle East, Russia, and China—but there was also another pattern, one that was potentially a circle of peace.

Years passed from the time of my dream. (We may have a vision or dream, but we usually don't wake up the next morning and pack our bags.) One day in 1986, I was absentmindedly spinning a globe that I kept in the corner of my trailer. I put my finger on the thirty-fifth parallel where I lived and whirled the globe. Twelve sites leapt out at me: the Santa Monica Mountains, where I lived in California; the Seneca Reservation in upstate New York, where Yehwhenode, an Native American elder woman lived; Spain; Italy; Greece; Israel; Palestine; India; Tibet; China; Siberia; and Japan. At that instant, I realized that this circle of countries formed the giant wheel of my dream. I knew immediately what I needed to do, and the World Wheel Project was born.

The first spoke of the World Wheel was in Malibu, California, not far from where I lived in retreat for five years in the Santa Monica Mountains. I needed to begin my work in my own region before I felt comfortable to involve other communities and cultures. Frank Lloyd Wright's family generously offered their land on a precipice overlooking the Pacific Ocean as a site for the sculpture and performance ritual. I came down every day to gather red, black, white, and gold stones on the beach with a friend, which we carried up the steep hillside in burlap bags. Using dirt, sand, and colored ocean pebbles, twelve friends helped me create an Earth Wheel, twenty-five feet in diameter, with a large upright lava stone in the center that stood five and one-half feet high. A circular fire pit surrounded the base of the center stone, symbolizing the harmony of male and female forces in our society. This creation was an act of prayer that we may find this harmony within our world.

The performance piece representing human origins began in response to my first question, "Where do we come from?" Androgynous beings emerged from a lake onto a sandy shoal at the site. As they peeled out of wet membrane skin-suits, they became a black man and a white woman. People with animal masks stood nearby, their visceral sounds puncturing the silence.

The next performance piece addressed my second question, "What is it that ails us, personally and communally, and how does this affect the planet?" Our sickness was depicted as the national arrogance of the United States, the misguided belief that we always know what is right for other countries. This "holier than thou" attitude has brought death and destruction to people and cultures around the world.

In response to my third question, "What is it that heals? What is the solution?" I appeared as Gaia, the earth silhouetted against the sky. My hair was woven in a tumbleweed, and my body and clothes were covered with mud. I looked directly into the eyes of each person, entreating them to come up the hill to the Earth Wheel and reconnect with the ancient wisdom that we are one living organism rather than separate isolated beings. Everyone danced late into the evening, a joyous affirmation of the unity of animals, plants, stones, and people—all creations as one earth family.

"Western Gateway" is the first sacred site of the World Wheel and is known as exceeding and expanding the boundaries of what we ordinarily think of as art and sculpture. Encompassing the environment as a whole erases the distinction between performer and audience and merges with life itself. This Earth Wheel in Malibu remains a potent touchstone for ceremony and celebration.

When Vijali left her studio life and her husband and sold all her earthly possessions, she became in essence a traveling artist-healer who carried with her only her tools and a photo album of her work. She got off airplanes in foreign countries with no plan, no money, beginning with only the names of some contacts. She met people, lived among them, and told her story; they invited her to a place to make a sculpture and ceremony. The locals accepted her immediately. They could see that her courage, commitment, skills, and focus on her calling—her sheer determination to be her authentic self—was pure. In many sites, women cried when they saw Vijali's photographs. She immediately knew where the stone was that she would carve with an ancient spirit to empower them again.

Vijali's environmental sculptures define sacred sites and are created with the assistance of each village. Before creating her healing art with each community, she asked her three questions. This connected her with that community more and gave her information about what needed to happen when she made her art installation. Her three questions changed. They became (1) What is our essence? (2) What is our sickness, our imbalance—personally, communally and globally? (3) What can heal this sickness, and what can bring us into balance? After she asked her three questions, Vijali spend many months carving each installation. When it was completed, she created a ceremony for healing, danced, and invited the community to participate. The performances held on the sites of the sculptures are a collaboration between Vijali, local artists, performers, and each host community. Through this process, the World Wheel provides a transformative experience for each community, addressing spiritual, social, and ecological issues while activating an awareness of the interrelatedness of all life.

Years after Vijali completed the first world wheel for peace, she had another vision to expand her first World Wheel to a second in the Southern Hemisphere. She is still making art and ceremony to heal, as well as expanding her process to include community action by helping local people build schools or medical facilities after her sculpture and performance.

We are incredibly inspired by Vijali and her wonderful work. She continues to expand her beautiful work after almost thirty years of creating environmental sculptures and altars for healing, peace, and compassion, while addressing the hopes and problems of communities all over the world through the arts.

Art truly transformed Vijali's life and the lives of all people she's touched. We know that not everyone can just give up everything or become an artist-healer. Each person will use art differently; each person is on a career path. But Vijali is an extraordinary testament to what finding your essence is all about—how to see yourself living your life to its fullest and make it happen; how to find your own unique, original healing journey. Vijali's story is about reflecting on your essence and your life to help you define your own purpose.

We encourage you to think about how you can use art not only to heal your own life but also how to bring art into your work as way of healing to help others—the focus of this week's praxis.

Vijali Hamilton, a stone sculptor and art activist for peace, tells about her sculpture for peace and working with native women in Senegal, Africa, in *The World Wheel Journeys*.
http://www.youtube.com/watch?v=pPx63pv07ok&list=PLMm-0ccB
-CYpmKktLEws7WlrNyNg2QDnu&index=7

## Week 9 Praxis

First, we have a guided imagery that allows you to go within yourself and discover a clearer image of your essence.

## *Guided Imagery: Finding Your Essence*

Relax and focus. Find a comfortable position and settle into your body. Take a deep breath, breathing into the area around your heart. Feel yourself relaxing and letting go of tension you may be holding in parts of your body. As thoughts come into your mind, simply notice them and allow them to float away, like clouds in the sky.

Focus on the experience of being spacious and grounded. Give yourself permission to have *this* experience, right here and now. You are exactly where you need to be in this moment. Now, in your mind's eye, see yourself in your body and see yourself in your life, doing things, having things. Watch yourself for a moment in your own life. Simply witness the person you are.

There is a part of yourself that watches you live your life in your body. This inner witness is your essence. Experience what it feels like to be who you truly are, without doing, without having—just being. Allow yourself to experience being alive in this huge spaciousness and in total freedom. Rest in this moment, be with yourself in your essence, and see who you are.

Now imagine you are sitting in a circle of friends who love you and support your healing work. This sacred, caring circle can be in a place you love in nature. It can be on Vijali's land where she lives now in Utah, a conference center, or a classroom—wherever you want it to be. Imagine that Vijali sits in front of you in a lotus position with flowers in her hair. Vijali looks you in the eyes, smiles, and asks you her three questions:

**"What is your essence?"**
- Allow your imagination to open up the possibility of this answer.
- You may hear a word or see a vision of yourself in action somewhere. You may experience a landscape, a place of being. You may see colors or experience feelings. Relax into this answer and just be patient.
- Return to the experience of your essence. Remember that there is no right answer—just yours.

**"What is it in your life that keeps you from being in your essence?**
- Allow the answer to come to you. What are your barriers? What are your obstacles? What are your fears, and what holds you back?
- Return to the place of your essence.

- Now that you have experienced your essence and have a sense of what those obstacles may be, how can you transcend them?

**"What do I need in my life to move through my obstacles, to reside and live from my essence?"**
- Just be with this for a while. Take a deep breath, focusing on the area around your heart. Grounding yourself, feel the chair and the floor. Allow yourself to be embodied in the place of your essence.
- Feel gratitude toward yourself for deeply connecting to your wisdom. Feel yourself connected to the earth. Now see yourself as your essence, without your obstacles, acting in freedom.

When you are ready come back, open your eyes and consider what you've been asked and what you've seen. As you reflect on the answers to these three questions, think about the last eight weeks. You have been on your own journey of healing with art for two months, making your own visual art, poems, dances, and music. You have also been writing in your journal, and you have been thinking about your final Medicine Art project and how to heal something in your life that calls out to be healed. Your journal and your work up to this point have been capturing your essence. Looking at your journal and at the art you have been making, what have you been doing? What can you glean about your essence from your creative work?

## *Medicine Art: Find Your Essence*

Next we will make art of our essence, obstacles, and healing. Place all the different art supplies, colored pencils, and collage materials in front of you. For the next hour of studio time, we will make art answering each of Vijali's three questions. Don't worry about what you will do; just have fun and make art.

You can use your guided imagery for images. If you saw something in your guided imagery that was completely different, that's perfect, too. Enjoy the expression of art and creation that you have right now. Remember, like all Medicine Art, there is no "right" or special way to do it. We did guided imagery to go deeper and connect with your inner image of your essence. You can make this Medicine Art any way you want to; you can even do the three questions on sequential days.

Open your journal. If the page is not large enough, get a bigger one if you need to or use more than one page. Either way is fine.

1. First, what is your essence? Draw for about thirty minutes or as long as you wish, like we do in our classes. You can begin by just writing one or two words and then start making art. Do what you want. There is no right or wrong way.

2. Next, what is holding you back? Draw whatever comes to you for as much time as you want. Again, you can also choose to follow your own pattern and inklings.

3. Finally, what do you need to do to heal? What art or spiritual practice will coax this essence from within you? Draw or write, working for the time you need to finish.

After you answer Vijali's three questions with Medicine Art, write what you experienced in your journal. Reflect on this process and who you are. Record what is happening to you in your life as you find your essence, obstacles, and solutions.

෨     ෨     ෨

The next step is sharing what you've learned about yourself, the ones you love, your coworkers, your community, and the world. Share your drawings, sculptures, writing, thoughts, feelings, and love with anyone in your art-healing community.

What can you do now to change and live your essence? You can keep working on your final Medicine Art project, change it, write a book, get a new degree or career, start a blog, make an art-healing club, set off on a journey, or, like Vijali, sell everything and make a pilgrimage to twelve countries to heal the earth. These are just a few examples of what people have done to take action in their life after they find their essence. We'll discuss this more in the next section, which continues with Samantha's personal story of art and healing.

## Samantha's Story: Finding Her Essence

As Samantha continued at the university, she became more and more successful at academics, but art and healing was put on the back burner. Her essence was eclipsed by work and proved difficult for her. Her essence was to be an artist-healer; her obstacles, her work and career; and her healing, going back to her essence. She told us how painting helped her find her essence again.

Painting outside in the streets helped me speak my truth where others would see it. I had space to express my discontent with a system that did not support my expression and forced me to conform to a certain methodology. I began to see my paint as a healing force that acted as friction against the machine that perpetuated woundedness in myself, others, and the earth. When I saw my art around the city, I could smile. Each smile helped me feel happy again and return to a sense of wholeness. I became less stressed by deadlines and pressure. I learned to accept myself and my talents. I released toxic emotions. I made new sacred relationships, and I created beautiful memories that can heal and impact others.

I realized that I became a participant in my own research study. I lived the experience of being healed through art. Through my own stories and stories of my research participants, I gained an immensely valuable insight into how art heals.

## Lessons from Samantha's Research Study

- Art helps students become clear about their needs, opening dialogue with parts of themselves that they are not aware of or are afraid of.
- Art as healing with others builds a sense of community, creates loving bonds between people, and helps illuminate the humanness in others.
- Art making helps process, alleviate, and integrate complex emotions such as anger, sadness, grief, anxiety, and fear.
- Art making helps students alleviate stress and promotes a sense of calmness and acceptance.
- When you heal yourself with art, you heal others around you.
- The quality of your art is not as important as the action of creating.
- Art serves as a reminder of the healing work a student has done, increasing retention of lessons learned.
- Art making can support new perceptions, fresh perspectives, deeper understanding, and integration.

This art and healing project helped Samantha become clear about her purpose and how important staying true to a practice is for emotional, physical, and spiritual health. "It helped me tune in to the importance of the subtle balance between the masculine and feminine forces in life. It brought me back to who I am at my core." Today Samantha continues to work proudly, fiercely, and with humility as an artist-healer, "knowing in my heart I am here to honor and heal myself, others, and the earth through the creative process."

 Samantha, a wall artist and student in Michael's class at San Francisco State University, tells how mural painting is a healing force for herself, other women artists, and the viewing public.
http://www.youtube.com/watch?v=meM_sGkNSiQ&list=PLMm-0ccB
-CYpmKktLEws7WlrNyNg2QDnu&index=6

## Summary of Week 9

- Do the guided imagery for finding your essence.
- In your journal, draw your essence, your obstacles, and what you need to heal to live your essence.
- Write about this experience in your journal.

# WEEK 10

# EXPERIENCING SACRED SEXUALITY

*Our body is our deepest expression of love—the tenderness of touch,*
*the empowerment of reopening, the intensity of union. It is a portal through*
*which we can become complete, experienced, loved, and loving.*

This week is about art and sexuality. Part of healing yourself is healing your sexuality. Sexuality is an important element in your life and contributes deeply to who you are. Psychotherapist Eric Maisel said, "If you bring your sexual impulses to your creative work ... you'll be working from deep in the genetic code, down where life wants to make new life and feel good in the process."[3] Healing your sexuality can be necessary for wholeness. It can also move you toward your own peak experience of sexual bliss, which is beneficial mentally, emotionally, physically, and spiritually.

Sexual healing is as individual as you are and very different for each person. It can be about simply celebrating sexual oneness; healing insecurity; healing fears; seeing and being your authentic sexual self; sacred sexual lovemaking; or healing sexual traumas like rape, incest, or sexual abuse. Women all over the world are using painting, dance, and theater to heal deep sexual traumas in programs and clinics. Whatever your story, in this week we will work with sexuality to help tie together the threads in this part of your healing journey.

---

3. Eric Maisel, *The Creativity Book: A Year's Worth of Inspiration and Guidance* (New York: Jeremy P. Tarcher/Putnam, 2000), 251.

# Healing Your Sacred Sexual Body with Art

Sexuality itself is an art. Mating rituals often involve elaborate dances and displays. We adorn our body to create an object of beauty. When we make love, it is a divine dance, a sacred movement. Our sexuality is celebrated. Our desire is the authentic longing of our soul to be known, touched, and loved.

The sexual acts of love are the most beautiful art forms. When you kiss, touch, and make love, you are participating in the most ancient sacred art form. Your dance, song, and adornment are all from the beginning of time. We make love in the embrace of the spirit lovers, the ancient beings who are the archetype of love. They are the first lovers; they existed before time and space in the stars, animals, and the breath of the earth. When we make love, we reenact their sacred worship and dance. We see our lover as the god or the goddess. We worship them as sacred.

Art has always been connected to sacred sexuality. Throughout history, artists have portrayed sacred sexuality in paintings, sculpture, and dance—from the *Birth of Venus* to the poetry of Rumi. Many religions believed that the union of female and male is a sacred marriage, a union of opposites that gives birth to forms. Sumerian, Greek, Egyptian, and Indian religions all celebrate the sacred union in art, poetry, theater, sculpture and ceremony. Tantra used the sexual union to achieve enlightenment; tantric artists portrayed the sexual union in beautiful paintings, sculptures, and temple architecture. In India entire temples are covered with carvings of couples making love, showing the sacred union of the opposites. The portrayal of sacred lovemaking was a doorway to spiritual ecstasy and peak spiritual experiences of enlightenment.

At its core, the most basic ritual is that of making love. Love makes anything sacred and holy, and it blesses everything. When we make love, we go deeply into visionary space where all the ancient legends are told to us. When any ordinary man or woman sees their lover as a god or goddess in their full beauty and magnificence on earth, they become the spirit lovers.

You can use art to heighten your experience of sacred sexuality and to share and enhance your own experiences of lovemaking, your body, and your sexuality. Every time you open your body for sexual union, you are becoming one with a Higher Power, as your body is the vessel of sacred love and divine sexual energy. Our sexuality is the desire of our spirit. Your mouth, penis, and vagina are all sacred portals for connection with your beloved goddess or god on earth. Our energy is attracted to the energy of the other. When we seek to love the beloved, we open ourselves physically, making ourselves ready for them to be with us. In orgasm, we sing the sacred music of the soul. We write love poems to our beloved to make the connection even more powerful.

What is so beautiful about our body is that it flows with the elements of the earth, since the body is the earth. We have the element of water in our blood and in our sexual fluids; we feel the fire of passion in the heat we make. When we make love, we create a connection to our creation from the elements. Sexual energy is the expression of the life force inherent in nature itself.

## Using Sacred Sexuality to Heal

Many people feel inhibited about their sexuality or deal with sexuality as a major issue in their lives. This can mean facing body-image issues, feeling unattractive, dealing with gender issues, or coping with trauma. Art gives you unbelievable freedom to express whatever sexual issues are in your life, no matter their degree. Making art does not embarrass, challenge, or hurt anyone or anything in your life. You are not strange or violent when you express sexual feelings in art. The paper can take it, the painting can take it, the journal can take it. Art can hold all unbarred expression for you. You have total freedom of expression to deal with who you are and what you feel.

Healing with art is experiencing the body as the beautiful container of our soul. Art integrated into sexuality is an opportunity to express what is hidden. Our sexuality is our most precious connection to intimately knowing ourselves and other human beings. The art of loving is the expression of who we are as humans.

Art and healing is an excellent way to deal with your sexuality, body image, desires, and loves. It is a wonderful outlet. You can make love poems of desire, write about who you are and what you want, and draw your sexual self. You can paint sexual self-portraits that free your goddess within, do body castings, make jewelry, or paint your body with henna. You can draw, paint, dance, and sing about your sacred portals, your connection to your beloved, and making love as sacred sexual union. Costumes, music, dance, drumming, smells, and scenes can all enhance your sexuality.

Art is a wonderful outlet for creating sexual ceremony, sexual environments, romantic settings, and even sexual theater. You can enhance your sexual life and move toward sexual bliss with art.

*A Sacred, Sensual Love Poem*

To my lover:
All I want is to completely surrender to you
in total sexual openness
This desire has saturated my life with love
My body is open to you
To make love to me
where ever and when ever
you want me
I trust you with the secret doorway
to love's deepest bliss

**—Anonymous**,
poem written in art and healing class

## Emily and Alyssa: Two Stories about Using Art to Heal Body Image

Emily, a young woman in Mary's class, had an aversion to her own body. She was afraid to expose herself. Every time she looked in the mirror, she found something wrong with her body. One day her hips were too wide; another day she hated the mole on her face. She was hypercritical and had a self-image of being fat. In the mirror she saw a distorted reflection of who she was. Emily realized that she was out of control and did not know what to do. She was uncomfortable and knew that she needed to heal her image of her own body.

For her final Medicine Art project, Emily asked her boyfriend to do a collaborative project with her. She asked him to take photographs of her, paint her, and make art with her body. She began by painting a mask on her face and asked him to take pictures of her in nature with silk fabric draped over her. Her objective was to create art and illuminate the beauty of her body. She wanted him to help her portray her authentic expression of herself and her sexuality, not a provocative false image. Through the photographs, she would see what he saw through his eyes.

The photographs he created were unbelievably beautiful images of her. She had never seen herself like that before. A tender yet strong trust emerged from the project, and they were able to take a step forward together in her life.

Emily was afraid to share the photographs with the group, so Alyssa, another woman in the group who was also afraid to share her body image, stood up to present. Alyssa said, "I hate my body." She went on and on about what was wrong with it. She was a beautiful woman and she was thin, but she also had a distorted body image. Her project was to do something to liberate herself from her fear. She stood in front of the group and took off her T-shirt. Underneath, she was wearing a black leotard.

She said, "This is my greatest fear. I will expose myself to you." She stood in front of the group in the skin-tight leotard. She shook with fear. What spontaneously happened next was a miraculous process. Every student received a reflection of her beauty. Then, in a beautiful ceremony, each person looked in her eyes and told her the beauty they saw in her. Alyssa stood, cried, and received the blessings.

It can be difficult to see, feel, and share your body and these deep feelings of sexuality with others. Mary told her, "Hold this space and receive these words. Let them go into your heart and know it is the truth." After Alyssa's presentation, Emily found the courage to share her beautiful Medicine Art project.

Emi, a teacher of Art as a Healing Force with Mary at the University of Florida, talks about loss, grief, and sexuality through art.
http://www.youtube.com/watch?v=eMD67bvEOyI&list=PLMm-0ccB
-CYpmKktLEws7WlrNyNg2QDnu&index=5

## Healing Trauma or Abuse

Healing with art is a very powerful tool for healing sexual trauma and pain. It has been used by survivors of sexual abuse or trauma and by art therapists for many years. It's powerful because art is explicitly vivid, graphic, and articulate in its process. The imagery you create when you make art is deeply personal, and you can go deeper into the memories of your body than in psychotherapy or guided imagery. Art can release the pain you hold. Art unlocks painful memories by opening your unconscious portals of creativity. In the total intimacy of your journal, paintings, and all your art, you can express rage, pain, and intensity without holding back.

If you have experienced sexual trauma, making art for healing sexuality can be very difficult, emotional, and dark, but you can handle it yourself. Maybe your friends can't take it, your therapist can't take it, or your family can't take it, but you can deal with it. You have been there and lived it and lived through it and it's over. Painting, dancing, poetry, and so forth can hold the graphic imagery. No one needs to see it but you. You can look at ugliness, despair, or outrage; that is powerful and healing. You can face what you feel most. There is nothing inside your body you can't handle because it's already inside your body. Letting it out into the light is your first step toward deep healing.

Art and healing is a powerful way to heal from a painful or traumatic event such as child sexual abuse, rape, and anything you remember that needs healing. Memories of trauma are one of the most basic human emotions. These memories can be from previous lifetimes, DNA, or even of another person. When people are violated, they are wounded, but sacred sexuality can never be taken from them. All people have a well-spring of sacred sexual energy that is as huge as their spirit.

### Artist-Healer Profile: Eve Ensler—One Billion Rising

*The UN now says that one out of three women on the planet will be raped or beaten in their lifetime. We're talking about the desecration of the primary resource of the planet.*

—Eve Ensler

Eve Ensler is a playwright, performer, and activist. She has taken art and healing to a level where she uses words and dance to heal violence against women. She is an inspiration to all of us who use art to heal. In her autobiography, *Insecure at Last*, Eve wrote about how she was raped and brutally beaten by her father, the CEO of a food company, from ages five to ten. Her sexual abuse experiences have been turned into art that heals women and the earth.

She is the author of *The Vagina Monologues*, an award-winning play that has been translated into more than forty-eight languages and performed in more than one hundred forty countries. Eve's experience performing *The Vagina Monologues* inspired her to create V-Day, a global movement to stop violence against women and girls. She has devoted her life to stopping violence, envisioning a planet in which women and girls will be free to thrive, rather than merely survive.

Today V-Day is a global activist movement that raises funds and awareness through benefit productions of *The Vagina Monologues* and other artistic works. In 2011 more than 5,600 V-Day benefits took place. To date, the V-Day movement has raised more than $85 million and educated millions about the issue of violence against women and the efforts to end it; crafted international educational, media, and PSA campaigns;

opened the revolutionary City of Joy community in the Democratic Republic of Congo; launched the Karama program in the Middle East; and reopened shelters and funded more than 13,000 community-based antiviolence programs and safe houses in the United States, Haiti, Kenya, Egypt, and Iraq. In 2001 V-Day was named one of *Worth* magazine's 100 Best Charities; in 2006 one of *Marie Claire* magazine's Top Ten Charities; and in 2010 one of the top-rated organizations on GreatNonprofits.

V-Day stages large-scale benefits and produces innovative gatherings, films, and campaigns to educate and change social attitudes toward violence against women, including the documentary *Until the Violence Stops*. It also holds community briefings on missing and murdered women in Juarez, Mexico.

Eve took the energy from *The Vagina Monologues* and V-Day and created One Billion Rising, a dance against violence to women. One Billion Rising is the largest art and healing event in history. It was the biggest mass global action to end violence against women and girls in the history of our species. One Billion Rising marked the beginning of a new world, ignited by a new energy.

On her website for One Billion Rising (onebillionrising.org), Eve has listed the huge dance ceremony's victories, including bringing together people, creating solidarity, waking up the world to violence against women, and making the best dance videos ever.

Keri, one of the students in Mary's class, performed *The Vagina Monologues* in Gainesville, Florida, as her final Medicine Art project. She was director, producer, and actress, and three students from the class were part of the play. They performed on V-Day at the local theater, and they put on an art auction of healing art done by the students in Mary's class. The money they raised—more than $5,000—went to Peaceful Paths, a local shelter for abused women. That is how easy it is to change the world and help prevent violence against women with art.

## Week 10 Praxis

### *Guided Imagery: Finding Sacred Sexuality*

Allow yourself to go to a place where you feel the essence of the rhythm of your heart and your breath. Imagine that your body resides in an infinite field of eternal love. Your beautiful body is the embodiment of this consciousness. Within this body is the beautiful, sensual, and physical state of being. This is a space where you are deeply connected to the source of your own sexuality. Within this sacred body is desire, yearning, and passion.

Connect with the rhythm of your own breath and the gentle pulsing of your own heartbeat. As you experience the embodiment of your essence, feel yourself residing in a perfectly designed body that holds your life and gives you the ability to unite in sexual union. Within this body, a physiological and anatomical construct is interfaced perfectly for you to make love. Being sexual is as simple as breathing. You open to the life force within. Connect with the intention to love, be open, and freely express yourself in your body. Allow the mystery of what is unknown to unfold into the creative energy of becoming, being, and being known.

Your sacred sexual body holds the incomprehensible mystery of life as it unfolds in each moment. There is wisdom in this body. There is eternal wisdom as it makes love, speaks, moves, and performs every action. This mystery of love unfolds in every moment. The incomprehensible synthesis of God flows through your being. In your sexuality, this energy comes into the light.

You and your sexual body are the god, the goddess, and the ancient spirit lovers. As you make love or yearn for your beloved, you are the god and goddess singing, dancing, making poems, adorning. See yourself in adornment. See yourself as the goddess, the god, the lovers of legend. Your body resides in an infinite field of life. Love opens a portal that allows you to channel this divine light, the healing force. Through making love, and through the creative process, you become illuminated, full of grace, and filled with feelings of healing. All of us are connected and healed within the moment of union. This sacred union is an illumination of grace.

Invite your sexual spirit to shine, to shift from ordinary to extraordinary. Allow the mind's chatter to simply flow away with your breathing. Experience the moments of vastness and silence as you feel the communion and expression of sexual essence. Within this extraordinary emptiness, allow your spirit to fill you up so you can become accessible to the greatest healing force. Resonate in this consciousness of your own being, feeling the connection between you and this infinite consciousness. Cultivate this experience of presence. Feel the vastness of this consciousness. This is a field of universal belonging. You have existed before the beginning of time, and you will exist until the end of time.

Return to your breath. Allow your breath to fill you, expanding your heart naturally. Imagine yourself embraced by pure light. This light has a sensual resonance that reverberates with a soft and subtle vibration. Feel this sexual energy. It is the life force. It is this energy you will experience for making love and when you vibrate with your inner healing force. You are in alignment with the life force. As you access the infinite within you, manifest it in your sexuality and connect with your beloved. It flows through both of you. In union you come into a place of pure light. In union you are connected to a life force greater than the two of you becoming one—a conduit for spirit to flow through you. The lovers heal deeply with this spirit energy. This is God's light on earth. The spirit lovers are the sublime manifestation of the highest level of consciousness, which is love.

## *Medicine Art: Draw from Your Guided Imagery about Sacred Sexuality*

Draw something you saw in your guided imagery. You can draw your sexual self, sexual energy, or erotic dreams. You can draw your sexual self connected to the infinite. You can draw the spirit lovers, the first archetypal lovers. Draw anything that you saw, dreamed, or glimpsed about yourself, your beloved, and your love. Here are some ideas based on what students have done in the past:

- Write love poems to your beloved.
- Paint your beloved.
- Paint making love.
- Make photographs or films to depict your love and your beloved.
- Make erotic art, paintings, sculptures, dance, and songs.
- Make theater, costumes, or scenes to intentionally enhance sacred sexuality.
- If you are pregnant, paint your belly with henna or washable paints to become the Earth Mother, seeing yourself as beautiful.

## *Guided Imagery: Healing from Trauma or Sexual Abuse*

This guided imagery is for people who have experienced sexual abuse, rape, incest, and other trauma. Unfortunately, many, many people have this experience. The guided imagery can be useful for anyone because most of us have experiences of sexuality that were uncomfortable or traumatic, and the guided imagery and art making that follows is very healing.

To begin the guided imagery, invite what protects you to come and be with you now. Make a sacred space where you are safe. Invite, call, and find your spirit guides, ancestors, spirit animals, teachers, and lovers to come with you as you go into this process. You never need to go alone.

Relax deeply. Slow your breathing. We will go together into a deep moment of remembering an event that needs healing. You can invite any moment, memory, or vision into your imagination. It can be a moment of abuse or trauma, something that happened in your family—anything.

When you arrive, first, be loved. Listen to who or what around you loves you the deepest. Even during this event, love and care came to you from what takes care of you and loves you always. This love may come from a distance, from above, or from another time.

To do this, find a moment when you know you were loved and taken care of. Find the most loving moment in this life or another. Find the person who loved you most. Be there fully. Reach for God, a Goddess, Jesus, Buddha, or Mother Mary; a lover, parent, grandparent, or faraway passed ancestor; a spirit animal, an angel, or a spirit guide. This is about being loved and feeling love. Look deeply into the person or being's eyes and see the love. Feel it flowing through you like syrup in your body.

Realize that even during what happened to you, you were surrounded by infinite and eternal love. If you want to or if it comes to you, feel compassion for the person who hurt you. This may be very difficult or it may feel natural. Do only what is comfortable during this guided imagery. If it feels hard, you can stop, be loved, and rest, going deeper only if you wish. Pray for your eternal lover to be with you always. If you can, speak to them, thank them, and be loved now and forever.

## Camilla's Story: Healing Childhood Sexual Abuse with Drawing

Sexual abuse stories often emerge unexpectedly in guided imagery or art to heal. People remember or are ready to deal with abuse when they make art in a loving and secure place. After twelve weeks of making art, sharing poems, and dancing together, a woman named Camilla presented her Caritas art project. No one knew her story. Up to that moment, she had spoken to no one in the group about her personal life.

Camilla was a quiet woman who spoke with a Spanish accent. She was middle-aged, worked in a bank, and lived with a roommate in the city. During the class, she had occasionally shared warm, compassionate comments to help people. We could see she was full of love and spirituality and ready to open her life to something, but we did not know what it was.

She began her presentation. "I want to share a book of my paintings with you." She opened a large beautiful book of drawings, touching it like it was a newborn baby. She spoke hesitantly at first, in a low voice like a child's. We could see tears come to her eyes. "This is a painting of my despair." She showed a painting of a woman huddled in darkness with black arrows piercing her body, mouth open in a scream, eyes closed, hands on the edges of the page coming toward her.

We knew what would happen next. We have been through this before many times in the years we have taught workshops, classes, and worked with patients. We know that in a group of about thirty women, three of four will make their art about child sexual abuse and will have the courage and trust to share this devastating art with the group, often for the first time. Many more women in the group will have experienced abuse, rape, or violence but may not want to share or make their project about this difficult topic.

"It was about a trauma I had," Camilla said. She started crying. She paused. A woman got up and hugged her softly. Then Camilla continued, "It was about being abused." A long pause. More tears. She then showed us a book she'd made. She said it was her healing book.

She told us about it in her own words.

My healing project was an important activity that I've never done before in my life. This project was full of mixed feelings that went from fear, anger, and disappointment to calm, harmony, peace, bliss, and freedom. At the beginning of the project, I asked myself a lot about what area of my life I should heal. I went deep into my heart and I decided to explore my emotional world, and suddenly the answer appeared as I wanted it to. The outcome terrified me because my heart told me that I have to heal a wound I had been carrying for more than twenty-five years. I'd never had the courage to share this painful event that happened to me with anyone.

At that moment, my world turned dark. I did not want to share my pain with someone. I asked God one more time to help me, so he sent to me Mary. She is a wonderful woman and the first person with whom I could open my heart. I shared with her the sexual abuse that I was victim of in my childhood.

My healing process started here. I had the courage to tell her all the suffering, fears, and distress that event in my life had caused. She gave me a strong emotional support. She cared for my heart and told me the right words for me to continue my healing process. She also advised me to make drawings where I could take out all the feelings this event could cause in me. This was extraordinary advice. Pencils, papers, and my willingness to heal myself were my powerful tools to heal my heart. Meditation and prayer were also important to heal myself.

Throughout my meditation, I asked the Superior Power to help me get out of the dark emotional world where I was living. My first image was the name of my healing process, which I titled *My Pain, My Sorrow, My Freedom*. This gave me a crystal-clear picture. I knew that I had to recall very painful memories, but through these memories, I was sure that I would find my freedom. During this healing process, I had to face a very difficult and painful time. It was not easy to recall those moments when I was abused. I cried so much. My body reflected all the feelings that I had in those negative moments. Many times I felt that I could not handle those burdens; however, I realized that the best way to heal pain is to face it. As a result, I decided to face my fears and go forward with this project. In my weakest moments, I prayed. I said to God, "God, this is the moment to take out all this pain from my heart. Please help me." I felt a great release after I prayed. Praying is undervalued to help people have the strength to go forward in their lives.

As I said before, drawings were very important in this healing project. I'd never imagined how powerful it could be to represent my feelings through drawings. Each drawing was a step that I walked on to move forward in my healing journey. After each drawing, I felt that my heart withdrew all the pain it needed to remove. This was a wonderful feeling because during the time I was drawing, I felt pain and I cried a lot.

All the steps in this journey were like a walk that showed me a world I hadn't known before. This is the world of art and healing. From my personal experience, I can tell you that art is the sweetest way to heal any kind of pain—emotional or physical. Now I can say that I am still working to heal my heart. Art helped me open my heart to a new world. I closed the cycle of pain, darkness, and sorrow. I was reborn. I am starting to write a new book in my life. The past has no power over me.

Camilla opened each page, and many women cried. Some got up and hugged her and thanked her for this courageous act of sharing. It could only have happened in a caring community with love and lack of judgment, in sacred space, where Camilla's guides and prayers could be with her as she faced her demons.

Art and healing creates this by itself. When you make art to heal in sacred space and look inside for what needs to be healed with the help of the ancestors, religious teachers, and a loving group of people who are intentionally caring, magic will happen. This is why art and healing is now being used by women to heal sexual abuse all over the world in clinics, outpatient programs, shelters, and hospitals. With this book, you can make art to heal yourself or with a therapist. Art heals.

**Lessons from Camilla's Story**
- Often, sexual abuse memories come during a guided imagery about what needs healing.
- You need a safe, sacred place to find these memories.
- Guided imagery has spirit guides, angels, God, and religious figures to help you see the darkness of sexual abuse.
- Telling someone you trust is a first step.
- Art is your tool to heal; it heals you by itself.
- Sharing helps you connect with a community of women.
- Images you draw, write about, dance, or sing heal more powerfully than you could have believed.

### Medicine Art: Draw from Your Guided Imagery About Sexual Trauma

If you have experienced sexual trauma, you can start to heal with art right now. Take out your journal or a sheet of paper and draw from your guided imagery about healing sexual trauma. Bring in spirit animals, guides, ancestors, helpers, and people who love you if the images are difficult for you. Draw whatever comes to you—no censorship; just let what emerges emerge. Remember that you are completely safe now. Nothing can happen to you here. If you feel a therapist would help as you remember and look into the darkness, there are many therapists who specialize in abuse. Feel free to work with someone if that seems necessary for you. You don't have to face this alone.

## Summary of Week 10

- Do the guided imagery to experience sacred sexuality.
- Draw, write, dance, and so forth from this guided imagery.
- You can also write love poems to your beloved or erotic love poems to enhance your sacred sexuality.
- If it is applicable to you, you can also do the guided imagery to heal from sexual trauma.
- You can also draw or journal from your guided imagery about trauma and healing.

# WEEK 11

# ART, HEALING, AND
# THE END OF LIFE

*In death, the incomprehensibility of ourselves is experienced in*
*letting go and going into the realm of pure consciousness.*
*May we know that all the love we have ever known is ours for all eternity.*
*We can take it with us as we cross to the other side.*

This week is your opportunity to deal with end of life, death, and dying. As you live more mindfully, you can move into facing and experiencing death with a deeper level of consciousness. You can creatively make art to consciously address the end of life, grieving a death, or facing your own fears.

Part of this process you have been engaged in has led you to this moment to expand your understanding about death and end of life beautifully. After the last ten weeks of making art to heal, you have cultivated an experience that allows you to understand what death is about. Throughout the book, we have changed your consciousness to create an opportunity to embrace the phenomenon of death with a deeper awareness. With this awareness we invite you to take this process to a place of extraordinary healing.

When we pay attention to death, we pay attention to something elusive and mysterious. When we make art around death, we access perceptions that are so subtle that we usually miss them. We can miss the subtle shift of consciousness that takes place around death. The experience of the time between life and death is ancient, mysterious, and powerful. Making art in or about this time can be extraordinary and life changing.

All the art you make in this twelve-week process moves you one step further in your awakening. This chapter is at the end of the book because this work is so powerful—dealing with death is focusing on your own true liberation and transcendence. As Elisabeth Kübler-Ross said, "For those who seek to understand it, death is a highly creative force. The highest spiritual values of life can originate from the thought and study of death . . . When I die I'm going to dance first in all the galaxies . . . I'm gonna play and dance and sing."[4]

From time immemorial, art has been used for dealing with death. In indigenous cultures, ancient cultures, and modern cultures all over the world, artists have created art about death and about people who have died. The art is made for many reasons. It is created to remember people who died and to access their wisdom. In Papua New Guinea ancestral masks represent specific ancestors and bring the spirits of the deceased back to the people. Those spirits share with the living the positive attributes they possessed during their natural lives. We make art to honor the deaths of warriors, chiefs, heroes, and heroines. Memorial art helps people remember culturally important people, what they stood for, and their accomplishments.

Most modern cities have statues, carved plaques, and even parks dedicated to people who have died. In Greece most temple art had the donors' names under the statues so they could be remembered long after their death. Japan's most sacred mountain houses art and tombs of people who died. Art is a way an ancestor or loved one can be seen, remembered, and honored. In Christian art, there are many paintings and sculptures, about the resurrection of Jesus. Michelangelo's *Pietà*, a statue of Mary cradling the dead Jesus, is emotionally moving and transformative for the viewer.

In ancient Greece, part of medicine was seeing death as a journey. The hospital in Delos, which had holistic and spiritual methods of healing along with herbs and surgery of the time, was directly across from the cemetery on the neighboring island of Rhenia. Patients could see the cemetery and be reminded of death every day, at every moment. When someone died, the dead person would be taken in a special boat across the straits to the cemetery for the burial ceremony. A marble sculpture was placed on the grave as a tombstone, along with carvings of the person and their family saying good-bye. Part

---

4. Elisabeth Kübler-Ross, *Death: The Final Stage* (New York: Touchstone, 1975), 1; "Kübler-Ross Free at Last," *Sydney Morning Herald* (August 24, 2004), http://www.smh.com.au/articles/2004/08/26 /1093518009727.html.

of the healing in the hospital was to choose life or death, keeping the choice clearly in view. People in the hospital could see the cemetery, think about death, think about what they needed to do to live, and make life changes to heal. This strengthened their intent to follow a healing regimen and change their lives.

These art and healing ceremonies around death continue today. For example, in Tinos, Greece, a small village on the island across from Delos, villagers re-enact the burial of Christ each year for Easter. In an evening service, they take a wooden life-sized Jesus down from the cross. The next morning women in the village decorate a coffin in the small church with flowers and put him inside. That evening there is a church ceremony. People light their own candles from the candles in the church that surround the coffin. The people pass under the coffin as if they are going under a bridge and take the decorated coffin out of the church to walk it through the small village in the dark night with their candles. They carry the coffin in a procession to each of the three small churches in the village.

All the villagers participate in this ceremony about death. As the flower-draped coffin visits each church, everyone goes under the coffin as it enters the church and under again as it comes out. The procession goes past each person's house. The children see the coffin decorated by their mothers pass each of their own houses. The whole village sings as the coffin is paraded down the small winding paths between the white houses. This intimate ceremony about death is very powerful. It is an art and healing ceremony, ancient and real. It involves art, decoration, music, and dance in sacred ceremony with the whole village, with people of all ages. For four whole days, the people are embodied with death. They touch the wooden statue of Jesus, touch and smell the flowers, and dance under the coffin over and over again like an ancient snake dance. They sing during this time, feeling, experiencing, and knowing death deeper than they did before.

The Mexican Day of the Dead, *Día de los Muertos*, also celebrates the dead. People go to cemeteries to be with the souls of the departed and build private altars containing the departed ones' favorite foods and beverages as well as photos and memorabilia. The intent is to encourage visits by the souls so the souls will hear the prayers directed to them by the living. Families make art, masks, poems, and plays for their departed ancestors. The famous painted skulls, dances, and colorful costumes honor the dead and are done with joy and even humor.

Art is now used extensively at end of life in hospice and hospitals and at home. Therese Schroeder-Sheker pioneered playing the harp at end of life to reduce physical and emotional pain and help a person have a conscious death. When we say "conscious death," we mean that the person is able to make the transition with peace, awareness, and acceptance, allowing the transition to be as natural as breathing. A conscious death is breathing through the moment when the body dies and the spirit lives on. Currently there are harp programs in many hospitals and hospices. Hospice has also used visual arts to make healing environments and put art, paintings, sculpture, and music in rooms for people at end of life. Storytellers write people's life stories to share with family, dancers, and poets who work in hospice and with people at home at end of life. Art changes the end of life experience completely. It is a powerful doorway to spirituality at a time when it is needed most.

Artists in Arts in Medicine programs do many projects with people at end of life. Shands Arts in Medicine at the University of Florida made a wall that has tiles from patients and families, many from end of life. The artists set up an open studio next to the cancer center for patients, families, and staff members to paint a tile. Each tile was then put on a large wall in the hospital atrium. Each person who enters Shands passes it before they reach the elevators. The tile wall is a beautiful project of art and healing. Each tile is reflection of the life of someone who was at the hospital.

This week we have provided many stories about how the arts can heal the pain of loss in our lives.

## Our Experience and Visions of End of Life

Both of us work with and think about death often and have our own experiences and visions of end of life. As a nurse, Mary has worked extensively with patients at the end of life with art and healing. She teaches a course in end of life at the University of Florida.

Around the time when my parents died, I felt a palpably thinner veil between the world of life and death. This is an experience I had many times when sitting at the edge of the bed with someone who was dying. As I sat next to them, listening to their breathing, I focused on my own breathing, centering on the still point within myself. At the same time, my consciousness would embrace their energy, connecting deeply with them as they were dying in their body. I would imagine merging my consciousness with their consciousness. It was a deep experience of profound silence. There were no words, just a fluid embodiment of connection of our consciousness and spirits blending. I experienced it as a spaciousness where time and space reside forever.

With this deep merging and blending, we would move toward death, evaporating into the pulsation of the human heart and the pauses between each beat. We would become pure energy within the embrace of the each other's spirit. We would explore the world between spirit and earth, surrounded by a landscape of transition with no horizons. I would share the journey as the spirit moved away from the body of the dying person I was working with.

In my imagination I could see a vision similar to the matrix of light in Alex Grey's paintings. I would hold the hand of the person who was dying while they walked to the edge of the physical world as we know it. Their light body was beautiful and translucent and would return to its perfection. They would move across the veil to another dimension, and I would wait to see if they would return. This was a practice of moving across the threshold of life and death. I could never see across the threshold, but I felt like the individual who was dying could see the other side. In their eyes was longing, desire, and anticipation of extraordinary beauty incomprehensible to me on this side. In this experience of sharing death with another, I realized that there is extraordinary beauty and awareness around death. I don't know how to explain it; it's incomprehensible. In death, I saw the miracle of living. Death is incomparable and beyond words when you look on the other side of the veil. It's unexplainable. When you look back to life on this side, it's as incomprehensible as the other side. We only live in this world within the limits of our mind.

When Mary's grandmother was dying, Mary drove an hour each week to see her. Mary brought her sketchbook, took photographs, drew, painted, and wrote poetry about her grandmother. Her grandmother had Alzheimer's disease and suffered from dementia.

My grandmother became the object of my desire as an artist. She was really important to me. In my grief, I spent time making art. As I drew, my pencil caressed her face on the paper. It was a very loving experience to be with her in this truly beautiful way. I was grieving from my experience of being with her and seeing her though the eyes of an artist and a painter. I was listening to her breath with the ears of a poet. I would go down and visit and just draw. Then I would go home and paint images of her. All through her death, I fully experienced the presence of her aliveness before she died. I experienced her life almost more powerfully than I had before. Of course, there is sadness in death, of wanting to be with her and missing her. I did four beautiful paintings of her in her last year. We all have opportunities to make the experience of death richer and more fully embodied.

We fulfill our life journey with this transition. Death is the transition between spirit and earth. The life journey returns to spirit. We return to the infinite field of belonging and love from which we came. In this transition of consciousness, many people have speculated that we travel on a beam of light with guides, family members, and spiritual beings who welcome us into the field of eternal love. Death is connected to movement as we take love across the membranes, leave earth textures and forms, and move into the space between molecules as we enter a new consciousness.

Michael has also worked with people at end of life with guided imagery and art. He worked with his wife and his mother as they were dying, using guided imagery, prayer, and visions.

When I am with a person who is dying, I see a hole around his or her death that allows a huge energy to pass in both directions, from earth to the other side and back, which important to us who are still alive. It looks to me like a vortex or whirlwind. I can feel a lot coming down to everyone. When my wife, Nancy, died of breast cancer in 1993, I experienced this energy.

I feel the same kind of huge energy and connection with the other side at a birth. At a good birth, I have seen everyone fall in love. We are all bonded and everyone gets very high on the energy. At a good death, I feel the same thing. I feel a lot of information coming down to everyone present; there I feel and see the possibility of huge personal growth for the person who dies and for everyone around them. I feel that you can get catapulted from where you are to a lot further along by the energy that comes across the membrane from the other side. When a person who dies becomes pure love or pure spirit before death, you can be given a gift of love or spirit. After the death, you are able to fall in love or embody spirit. This gift comes to you from the dying person and from the situation as they cross the membrane.

Why is art and healing so good at helping people deal with death? Art has always been a way for people to see across the membrane into mystery, to glimpse other worlds. Art and healing can help you see a new positive imagery that re-storys a death. As you make art, you deal with emotions and release attachments. Art and healing are a natural way to deal with death. Crossing to the inner world to make art is slipping through a veil, almost like a small death. You die for a moment in your ordinary world of textures and forms and enter your inner world and the world of visions and spirits. That is like death. That is why art and healing help people use their creativity and inner vision to explore unresolved issues of grief. Healing unresolved grief is valuable. People celebrate life and their loved ones by making art about death.

## Michael's Story: Playing Guitar for Nancy as She Died

When my wife, Nancy, was dying of breast cancer, our younger son, Lewis, would serenade her for hours. She was in a liver coma from liver metastasis and was starting to lose consciousness. It was slow and gentle but totally real. Lewis was sixteen years old, and Nancy had been sick since he was twelve. One month earlier, the metastases in her liver and lungs had grown rapidly. Her two physicians had set up a special meeting to tell her. They met in an office across from the hospital so that neither would be alone with this woman whom they had learned to love during the four years they had taken care of her. When she heard the news, she did not cry. She looked right at them and her only reaction was to ask if she could still go to England to visit some English gardens. She had planned the trip for the whole spring and it was one thing she looked forward to deeply. I could see them both roll their eyes and look away. Then her medical oncologist, Sam Spivak, paused. "Of course you can, Nancy," he said, so gently. Later, I heard that he told a friend that if *he* were to die, he would just as soon die in an English garden.

Nancy not only survived the trip but also was not impaired during it. She ran through the gardens, sometimes two or three a day, her bald head covered with a hat. A raincoat protected her from the damp English spring. In a strange way, she was deeply at home, her face radiant and at peace. Her spirit was free. Once, I saw her sitting on a bench at the end of a long path of hedges. You could see the light around her rising. It was so beautiful.

When she returned home, her body rapidly became more ill. Her liver function tests were very high and she started to fall asleep and wake up alternately. Like usual, she did not want to know how long she had to live, but she wanted to make plans so that her children could be with her. She did not want Rudy, our older son, to travel away from home as he was planning to, so she asked me to call Sam and ask him if Rudy could go on a trip. Lewis was in the living room when I called Sam. He understood what I was asking Sam and why. He had been through this kind of call before. On the phone, Sam told me that Rudy should not leave, even for a week. I hung up and told Nancy that Sam had said that Rudy could not travel. Tears came to her eyes, which was exceedingly rare. The night before, she had told me that her relationship with Lewis needed to be healed. He was a teenager, and she had had trouble talking closely to him as she was dying. Now she needed some resolution, but she didn't want to discuss death. She paused. Lewis came up to her, kissed her, and said, "I love you, Mother." That was unusual for him, too. I could see her body loosen up and open and her spirit rise. It was like a weight had been taken off her. She had her resolution.

The next day she went upstairs into our loft overlooking the ocean and the mountains, never to come down again alive. She went into our bed where both boys had been conceived, nursed with love, read to, and sung to as babies. She started to hold a sacred beingness. Rachel Remen, in her book *Kitchen Table Wisdom*, called Nancy's state before her death "Sitting Dashan," the state in which a guru gives gifts to her followers. When Nancy's best friend, Elizabeth, came, she said that Nancy had turned into pure love. She had. Her personality had departed, and in its place was her eternal soul. She would only say to each person who visited her, "I love you so much. You are so beautiful. I am so happy to see you." She gave each person the gift of love as they came to pay their last respects and say good-bye.

Meanwhile, Lewis and Rudy made healing art, each in his own way. Rudy dug an enormous fish pond next to Nancy's English garden. He made garden art for her. It took his whole body and all his physical energy. He dug in the earth like he was making a huge grave. He would dig and then come upstairs and sit and tell stories with his mother; when she fell asleep, he would go down and dig some more.

Lewis had his own rhythm. He would go downtown, surf, and then come home and sit next to Nancy's bed whether she was asleep or awake, and he played his guitar. He was writing a soft, slow piece for her death that was so beautiful. I think it came right from his heart or even somewhere far deeper. He worked on the song and played to her throughout the days as she looked at him, had visitors, slept in her coma, and dreamed.

His guitar piece grew and was like a endless round; it caressed you like the wind. It encircled your body like Nancy's love, carrying you and making you feel taken care of, blessed, and in the hands of a greater force.

It was an acoustic guitar, soft and caring. Lewis just sat and played it for hours. And as his mother dreamed, she drifted with him, and he carried her. She floated on the music, and he cared for her perfectly in her last days on earth as his mother.

**Lessons from Michael's Story**
- It important for people at end of life to talk to their family about unresolved issues.
- Dying at home can be very beautiful.
- Guitar or harp music at the bedside of a person at end of life is soothing, spiritual, and wonderful.
- Music carries a person home.
- Death can take a person to love, to achieve the most spiritual moments of their life.
- A conscious spiritual death is healing to the person and everyone around them.
- Art allows family and fiends to participate in the death in an active, spiritual way.

## What You Can Do to Use Art and Healing with Death

There is a lot you can do in your life now to deal with death. If you have a loved one who is dying, you can make art with them. You can help make the place where they are sacred with art, altars, and music. If you are musician, you can play the guitar or harp with patients at end of life. You can volunteer in a hospice as a healing artist to work with dying people. You can make art to celebrate the love of a loved one or a revered figure who has died. You can help your own grieving process by making art about a loved one's death. Don't look away or abandon someone who is dying. Make art with them.

Making art and healing about death is a very healing way to help you grieve. It embodies death, bringing you into it and it into your body. Making a slide show or scrapbook of beautiful images, writing about a death in your journal, and telling the story of the death to friends changes your memories about the death of a loved one. It can re-story the death into beauty.

# Week 11 Praxis

## *Guided Imagery: Dealing with End of Life and Death*

Close your eyes. Center on your heart. Breathe slowly. Each time you breathe, relax and let your body soften. Feel your body melting into a place of complete openness. Take a few moments to be centered and imagine yourself becoming more and more open and relaxed.

Imagine your physical body in space and time. In your imagination feel your hands, arms, head, neck, and your entire torso, down to your toes. Feel the density of your physical body.

Now, in your mind's eye, imagine a figure of light approaching you, a translucent figure that is pure light. See the figure reaching out to you. This figure is a companion to take you to the other side. See yourself as a light being moving out of your physical body with your body resting below. Understand deeply that you will return to your physical body after the guided imagery. Now look back and see your body in a relaxed state of meditation, knowing you will return.

In your mind's eye, look forward. Look around. The landscape may be unfamiliar. You may or may not see a horizon. There is a veil of light, a soft shimmering curtain. Your guide opens the curtain, and you walk across to the other side. You hear beautiful music. The sound is soft—the most beautiful sound you've ever heard. As you look around, there is the most beautiful light you have ever seen. The figure stays behind the veil as you walk forward. Your light body dissolves into an infinite field of love. You are totally expanded in a field of consciousness. In this field there is a oneness with everything and a deep sense of peace. As you look around, recognize others. They are waiting for you with open arms. Allow yourself to merge with this experience, feeling yourself dissolve into pure spirit. Dwell in this place of light and simply feel the essence of being. There is no time, no forms—just an extraordinary sense of eternal peacefulness. Feel the pulsation of the spirit world. This place has breath and a heartbeat. You merge with it in this universal field of sacred love. Stay here as long as you like. Be open, simply be in peace, and breathe. Experience the eternal nature of the infinite field of love.

When you are ready, you may return, slipping through the veil. Your guide is waiting for you. As you walk across the landscape, see your body resting below. As you walk to your body, observe it with eyes of gratitude and deep appreciation. Now simply move back into your own physical body, reconnecting with your own physical heartbeat and breath. Feel the density of being back in your body. Feel the sensation of having skin, eyes, and a mouth. Your senses bring in the textures of being in this body in the physical world. In this moment, before you open your eyes, connect with your heart. Feel gratitude and appreciation for this body that holds your soul. When you are ready, open your eyes.

### Medicine Art: Draw from Your Guided Imagery about Death

Take out your journal and draw what you saw. As usual, you can draw anything you saw or anything that came up for you in the guided imagery. You can also write a poem, write in your journal, dance, and even sing or tone about the death imagery that came up for you. To give you some examples, the following are some powerful journal projects to consider. These ideas are based on what others have completed to change their lives.

- Write about what you would think or do if you were going to die in this moment, an hour from now, a week from now, a month from now, or a year from now.
- Write about your fears of dying.
- If you had a year to live, what would you do with your life in this year?
- Write your obituary as if you had died right now.
- Write your obituary as if you died at the end of a long life.
- Write about an experience of being with someone who died.
- Write a letter to someone who has died, such as your mother, father, or grandmother.

### Medicine Art: Making Medicine Art Projects about Death

- Play the guitar or harp with someone who is dying.
- Volunteer at a hospice as a healing artist.
- Make a scrapbook about the life of a loved one, family member, or revered teacher who has died.
- Write the life story of someone who is dying before they die.
- Interview a loved one close to death about their life.

- Make a film about someone at end of life or photograph them.
- If someone has died, go back in their life and create book of memories with photographs, objects, and so forth.

## Summary of Week 11

- Complete the guided imagery about dealing with death.
- Draw from your guided imagery about death.
- Journal about your thoughts about death.
- Using art, work with someone who is dying or at end of life.

# WEEK 12

# YOUR FINAL PROJECT AND TRANSCENDENCE CEREMONY

*It is true; we are more than we'd ever thought possible.*
*It is true; the beauty of the greatest light in the universe shines from within.*
*The greatest gift we give is the essence of our life and being.*

### Part One: Art and Healing Is About Experiencing Transcendence

Transcendence is the feeling of deep oneness and connection with something larger than we are. For us, transcendence is the goal of the art and healing process. Transcendence is the experience of the illumination of your soul or spirit. It means seeing yourself illuminated, beautiful, and full. As Alex Grey said, "The infinite vibratory levels, the dimensions of interconnectedness are without end. There is nothing independent. All beings and things are residents in your awareness."

As we brought up in the introduction, transcendence is the final theme in the Spirit Body Healing research study of how art heals. It is the conclusion of the research study and the conclusion to this book. Making spirit visible through an experience of transcendence is deeply healing to body, mind, and spirit. Spirit heals by being seen. In the art-healing process, glimpses of God or angels that participants may have had in the beginning of their healing journey grew immensely in power and meaning. People who have made art to heal have experienced the power of the universe, felt the presence of a higher consciousness, and often heard the voice of God or a Higher Power. They felt they had emerged into another dimension of great power and beauty where everything was illuminated. This is the goal of our twelve-week program. We want you to see your own spirit illuminated. It is both that simple and that complex at once. The experience of seeing, feeling, and smelling your spirit illuminated is a full experience of being. It is a moment of perfection embodied. It is a deep inner and outer healing experience.

The participants in the research study of how art heals often described hearing a message from a higher consciousness. Because messages from a higher consciousness can be associated with being crazy, people are initially reluctant to share the experiences with us. They had to trust that we would honor them and listen with an open mind. But the experiences were so powerful, they had to be shared. In excitement, joy, and love, people told us their stories, just as we have shared our stories of our twelve-week process in this book.

Don't be afraid if you hear the voice of a higher consciousness or see angels when you heal with art; it's normal. Many people who complete the art-healing process have this experience, and they are all people like you. For us, it is part of the process. When you make art to heal, you glimpse powerful, archetypal, and ancient images from the universe. For example, one day, we did a mandala workshop at Shands Arts in Medicine with eight women who had breast cancer. Mandalas are powerful circular art forms that bring wonderful balancing energy. Six women in this workshop drew angels in their mandala. None of them saw the others' mandala, and we said nothing to them about angels, transcendence, or even spirituality. The angels came to them in the mandala form in the simple act of art making. This experience of transcendence was deeply healing for all involved.

## Alex's Story: A Vision of Transcendence

Alex Grey is the most visionary artist-healer of our time. He is our culture's version of a Renaissance master painter. Alex sees deeper into visionary space than any other contemporary artist.

Alex was trained as an anatomical artist and worked as a medical illustrator drawing blood vessels, nerves, and organs. An incredibly skilled renderer, he moved on from this medium and became a performance artist, experimenting instead with multimedia art. Next, he and his wife, Allyson, had a series of visions of the spiritual nature of humans. After the visions, Alex made a series of paintings of the human body, all life-size. The images are etched on a mirror and framed with sculpture. The series starts with the body of three women and three men (one each Caucasian, African, and Asian) and then moves to depictions of organs, bones, blood, nerves, chakras, energy, and finally pure light. As discussed earlier, in week 5, this series is called *Sacred Mirrors*. It is made to be interactive, with the viewer standing in front of each mirror painting and seeing their own reflection merge with the image in the painting.

Seeing *Sacred Mirrors* is a transformative art and healing experience. It transports the viewer from ordinary space to sacred space, from body to illuminated spirit. Alex and Allyson have spent most of their lives building a temple for the sacred mirrors so people can visit to have healing, transcendent experiences. The temple is their huge lifetime art and healing project. Alex told us about the vision of transcendence that changed his life.

> My wife and I lay together and closed our eyes. We saw visions as one. One of the first visions was of a mind lattice—a realm of complete interconnectedness between all beings and things, via a love energy that was in an infinite, omni-directional grid, a sort of fountain drain, a toroidal shape. Each being and thing was one of the cells interlocked in this ongoing network. There was no reference point to the external world or external reality—it was all in the energetic realm and felt like the total bedrock of reality. This was the scaffolding of creation that the dreamlike world of mundane manifestation was draped over. It felt like a veil had been stripped away and I was seeing the way things really were. It was beyond time. It changed my entire point of view about what we are.
>
> I came back from that experience and looked at Allyson. She had seen the same transpersonal space at the same time. That just drove it home to me. I'm not saying that's it or that's the only space. But it was my initiation into a mystic headspace that I feel is profoundly true.

Alex and Allyson Grey share their transcendent visions with us so we can see our spirit illuminated. Like ancient artists in Tibet who painted the Buddha so that people could glimpse enlightenment, Alex paints transcendent visions so we can see the truth about how the world is made. We can see ourselves as light beings.

One of Michael's first experiences with art and healing involved Alex's art. Michael was working with a man who had terminal cancer and knew he would pass soon.

Michael was working with him to help him see across to the other side and move back and forth freely in visionary space. Together, they would do guided imagery exercises to move from the physical to the spiritual.

 World-renowned artist Alex Grey talks about visionary sacred art. http://www.youtube.com/watch?v=fM8zYUNBD3o&list=PLMm-0ccB -CYpmKktLEws7WlrNyNg2QDnu&index=5

One week the man brought Michael one of Alex's paintings, *Transfiguration*. The man was excited and full of life. It was as if he had awakened from a dream and was now balanced and holding a calm energetic power. He said,

> Look at this painting. I found it last night. This is the truth for me now. This is what I actually see when I do guided imagery with you. This is what I am seeing in my dreams at night. This is what the structure of space actually looks like to me now. The lines and points of energy are real. This is the truth for me now, as I am about to die.

Michael saw dramatic change in this man he was working with. He understood that the vision Alex had painted was what this man saw. The validation and clarification of the sacred, transcendent vision was deeply healing beyond words. When a visionary artist paints visions of transcendence and shares them with us, we are all healed.

We highly recommend visiting Alex and Allyson Grey's Chapel of Sacred Mirrors outside of New York City. You can have this life-changing experience and feel for yourself how art heals. Alex and Allyson perform sacred ceremonies to heal with art. Their whole lives have been changed by this vision; they are healing art in action.

> Allyson and I like to say that art is our religion. Art is the oldest living religious tradition and embraces all sacred paths. Every great wisdom tradition has manifested sacred art in many disciplines—paintings and sculpture, architecture, performance, dance, music, wisdom writing, and poetry. We believe that every day is a good day when we paint.

**Lessons from Alex's Story**
- We can see pure spirit.
- We can see spirit illuminated.
- We can make art of what we see.
- We can see interconnectedness and experience it as the truth.
- Art is a way for us to see and share this vision to heal ourselves, others, our community, or the earth.

## Guided Imagery: Experiencing Transcendence

Make yourself comfortable. Uncross your legs and arms. Close your eyes and let your breathing slow down. Take several deep breaths. Let your abdomen rise as you breathe in and fall as you let your deep breath out. As you breathe in and out, you may have feelings of tingling, buzzing, or relaxation. Let those feelings increase. You may feel heavy or light. You may feel your boundaries loosening and your edges soften.

Now let yourself relax. Let your feet relax and then your legs. Let the feelings of relaxation spread to your thighs and pelvis. Let your pelvis open and relax. Now your abdomen relaxes. Allow your belly to expand—do not hold it in anymore. Your chest relaxes, and your heartbeat and breathing take place by themselves. Let your arms relax, followed by your hands. Now relax your neck, head, and face. Soften your eyes. See a horizon blackness for a moment. Let these sensations spread throughout your body. Let your relaxation deepen. If you wish, you can count your breaths, your relaxation deepening with each exhale.

Imagine that you are in a place that is holy or sacred for you. It can be a church, a temple, an ancient ruin, a mound, a stone circle, or a wonderful place in nature like a waterfall, a mountaintop, or a sacred river. You can even picture a place where a person who is sacred to you has had a vision, such as the mountain where Moses saw God, Lourdes, Jerusalem, Mecca, or the tree Buddha sat under. Sit for a moment, absorbing the energy of this place. Feel all the people who have prayed and had visions before you. Feel the energy of the air, earth, water, and fire. See the visions of those who have come before you.

Look around you. The light is expanding and opening. Feel how the light radiates from within. This light is light itself, not a reflection of the sun. This light is divine light.

Now ask for a vision to come to you. It can be a vision of a deity you believe in, a religious figure you revere, a place in nature where you have had powerful experiences, a teacher, a loved one, an ancestor, or whatever spiritual vision you have had in the past that holds the most power.

The vision will appear all around you, out of time and space. It may come as a presence, vision, voice, light, or thought. When you are aware of the presence, listen to what comes to you. Receive the blessings, healing, support, love, and message the vision brings. Feel the knowledge of truth and power the message has. This message will change your life forever.

Rest in the beauty of the vision. Realize that you can have this experience again, whenever you wish.

## Medicine Art: Bringing in the Light

This is a Medicine Art project to bring the light into your body, mind, and spirit. It is a healing dance, like an ancient ceremony. We have done this all over the world, on sacred sites, in nature, in the center of medicine wheels. We invite you to do this, too.

Find a place in nature that is sacred for you. It can be a beach, a clearing next to a beach, a hilltop, a mountaintop, a mound, or a stone circle—anyplace you go that is sacred to you. You can do this exercise alone or with another person. If you choose to work with another person, stand apart, look at each other, and do it together.

Stand in the sacred place and pause. Give thanks for being there; give prayers for this special place. Close your eyes. Put your arms at your side and relax. Open your eyes. Now slowly—very slowly—raise your arms up on each side of your body until they are over your head. Touch your hands together at the top, as though you are pointing upward to heaven or the sun at noon. As you raise your arms, see the light from the earth getting brighter and brighter. You are creating a sacred dome of light around you. The dome of light rises when your arms are together at the top. Now slowly bring your hands apart and down to each side. This makes the light even brighter and brings it down over you and the earth, holding it there.

Stand in the light and feel its beauty and brightness. It is God's light on earth. You can bring in this light whenever you are healing. See a face in the center of the light. It is the face of a spiritual figure you love. It can be God, the Blessed Mother, She Who Gardens Us from Above, or She Who Loves Us.

## Part Two: Completing and Sharing Your Final Medicine Art Project

This is the last week before your project presentation and journal sharing. This final chapter is about *you*. In this week, you will complete your final Medicine Art project and present it. You can present it to yourself by writing in your journal a short description of what you wanted to be healed, what media you used, what the process was, and what it felt like. You can share your project with someone you love, or you can share it with an art-healing group. You can share it on the internet if you are working with a caring community there.

For this week, we will also share some more stories about final Medicine Art projects, what projects people made to heal, and what their sharing was like. When we do the Art as a Healing Force process as workshops or classes, twenty to forty people do it at once. At the end, in the final weeks, they present their final Medicine Art projects to the group in a deeply sacred sharing. Each person presents for about fifteen minutes; if it is a class, they also write a two-page explanation of what their project healed and how they did it. For forty people, it takes two whole days to share. The projects each are so beautiful. It's two days of crying, laughing, being in love, and feeling the beauty of art healing the human soul.

### *Final Project: What to Heal, What Media to Use, and What Process to Follow*

As far as your final project is concerned, by now you should be on your way. If you have your project already, keep working. If you have not decided what to do yet, we've put together some examples to help get you going. Then, after this, we have included many examples of what other participants in our university classes and in the Arts in Medicine programs across the world have done to help heal themselves, others, their communities, or the environment.

### *Working on Yourself*

First, imagine what you want or need to heal, for personal empowerment and growth or for a physical, emotional, mental, or spiritual illness.

- Physical illness: stomach problems, skin problems, cancer, any disease, chronic or acute illness, weight loss, depression
- Abuse history: sexual abuse, rape, violence
- Sexual concerns: experiencing sacred sex, gender, body image
- Spiritual growth: visions, Kundalini experiences, finding your essence
- Inner critic: put them in a box
- A death in your life: loss of an unborn baby, mother, grandmother, teacher, guide; help to grieve
- A relationship to grow, solve, or grieve: boyfriend, girlfriend, lover, father, mother, husband, wife, children, family, relationships
- Your environment: a healing garden, redecorating your bedroom or house
- Something you've always wanted to do: cook, paint, garden, travel, make a pilgrimage

## Jen's Story: The Art in Arthritis

Jen was a psychologist who suffered from severe rheumatoid arthritis. She had deformed joints, and her hands and knees and feet were swollen. She was in chronic pain and had difficulty moving. One day she arrived at Michael's office laughing and almost dancing. She looked completely different—much younger, more beautiful, and full of energy.

She was carrying a package and said, "I want to show you something." Jen opened the box and unrolled a painting on the table. It was a beautiful painting of a woman lying on the ground. The point of view was from above and behind the woman's head. You could see the top of her head, her body going away from you, and her knees apart and up. From between her legs, you could see the earth coming out.

I asked her what it represented to her. She said, "I am lying in the sun. My legs are apart, and I am giving birth to the earth. The whole earth—the continents, the oceans, the clouds, and the sky—are coming out of my vagina. When I painted this vision, I knew I was healing. I felt such huge energy and interconnectedness, such love come out of me that I know something radical had happened."

Jen was in fact healing. She'd had fewer flare-ups of her rheumatoid arthritis that had kept her in chronic pain for years. Her arthritis was healed. Jen had repeated surgeries to repair the deformities and has been much better for years. She moved, got a new job, bought a house, and made a new life for herself after having these visions of connectedness and oneness.

## *Working with People*

If you know someone who has breast cancer or some other disease, make art. You can be the artist-healer who helps them start their journey.

- Mother, father, sister, or brother with physical or mental illness or loss
- Family member who is disabled or has special needs
- Patients in hospital, older people, cancer patients, AIDS patients, and people in schools, prisons, and neonatal centers
- Art for recovery programs that need volunteers (find them on Society of Arts in Healthcare website or Google)
- Start a new program anywhere, such as hospital waiting room or atrium, community program, YMCA, veterinary clinic, or church

Start with your pain and theirs and move to where it goes. Paint, draw, write poetry, journal, make sculpture, mold clay, play music, dance, do theater, or create a ceremony. You can paint the other person, draw them, or invite them to make art with you. Play music on your iPod if you are in the hospital and make your room an altar. Bring in things that are sacred to you such as religious items or sculptures of spirit animals. Bring in paintings and photographs you love and hang them on the walls. Make your room an art gallery. Call in ancestors, spirit guides, and angels; invite them to come and be with you.

Do guided imagery, too. Diane Tusek's audio of guided imagery is wonderful, but you can do any guided imagery. This will relieve fear, side effects of treatment, and pain, and make you happier and more comfortable. Know you can heal; know you can feel better and make a new life.

## *Each Person Is Different*

The most important thing to keep in mind when you're working as an artist-healer with a person with cancer or any other illness is that each person is different. Each artist-healer is different, too. How can you possibly do the same thing with each patient? Dr. Lawrence LeShan, a psychologist who worked with cancer patients, said that it's abuse to work with patients and do only one therapy for all. That neglects the individual, or their "soul frequency," as health futurist Leland Kaiser would say.

We tell the artists and healers we work with to leave their agenda at the door and let what happens happen. If you have art supplies, will you make art? What if you walk into the room and the person does not want to make art but they want to sing? What if you are a painter and they want to be held, not make art? What if they want to throw you out? What if they want to tell you their story? What if they want to be with their children? Listen, look, love, and do what comes to you in the situation you are in with the person you are with. When you work with a person with cancer, go in and let magic happen with *no* agenda. Spirit will come and heal. Expect surprises. Invite a totally new and unknown magical healing to come, and it will—always more beautifully than you could have imagined.

We are artist-healers. Remember what an artist is. Artists are creative. They're new in every moment. Each work is different. The healing images are from the source. You are different from other people. The artist-healer is a new figure in healthcare and in art.

## Tips on Working with a Person with an Illness

Let's say you have a friend or loved one with cancer or a physical illness and you want to work with them as an artist healer. What do you do?

- Love them. Pray for them. Picture them in your mind's eye healed and strong. Love heals.
- Encourage them to make art. They can collage or write a poem with no rhyme. Art heals and brings miracles. Make art with them, draw them, sing to them.
- Encourage them and help make their world beautiful. Bring art, paintings, music, and videos to them. Decorate or help them beautify the space they are in. Make the space so sacred that you gasp. If it's appropriate, build an altar. It is important for someone to experience something beautiful each day. Beauty heals.
- Encourage positive re-storying or reframing of their situation, prognosis, and life now. Everyone can have a miracle and a good quality of life. Everyone can be healed—not always cured, but healed.
- There is tremendous power in hope and faith.
- Allow the person to express their pain and suffering in darkness as well as their gratitude and joy. It's not bad for them to cry. Be with them while the emotions are released. This is good. Speaking about death and fear is good, too.

- And as a friend, not an artist-healer, help them put together a healing pie of tools to address their basic self-care needs: diet, exercise, herbs, *qi gong*, or alternative healing—anything they are naturally attracted to.
- Do guided imagery with them, bring them tapes, and recommend guided imagery therapists.
- Encourage them to use creativity to express their spiritual life, honoring what is most sacred and precious to them.
- Try Diane Tusek's guided imagery CDs and audio files or other guided imagery you enjoy.

## Working in an Arts in Medicine Program

Remember that this final project is about healing yourself, others, your community, or the earth, and working with people as an artist-healer is a powerful way to do so. You can set up (or work in) an Arts in Medicine program in a hospital, school, community center, retirement home, prison, or church. It can be a big life change, like a career change or lifestyle choice. It is sacred work, a meditation. For some people, it's a dream come true.

It's a growing field too. Research on the healing effects of art with illness demonstrates why art and healing is used in hospitals for healing physical illness. All illnesses involve the body, mind, and spirit. Art and healing work by resonating with all three. It changes attitudes, which profoundly affects symptoms of pain and chemotherapy side effects. Art and healing promote hope and spirituality, which has been shown to promote physical healing.

Art and healing is now used with breast cancer patients in most cancer centers. There are Arts in Medicine programs that bring art to women with breast cancer. Breast cancer patients have made quilts, paintings, and altars to heal. Hollis Sigler, a painter, painted a large series of paintings about her experience with breast cancer; the collection toured many museums and hospitals. Art is powerful for women with breast cancer and for their families.

To work in a program, find a place that calls to you. Look online. Search for art and healing programs in your local community using key words like *hospital*, *Arts in Medicine program*, and the name of your city or closest city. Call them and offer to volunteer.

If there are no programs in your town, it's time to start one. Maybe you're the one to do it. Many students in our twelve-week process have started their own Arts in Medicine program in a retirement home, school, or hospital.

**Artist-Healer Profile: Annette Ridenour—Creating Healing Environments**

When you go into San Diego Children's Hospital, you see huge dancing sculptures, movable art at a child's height, and beautiful rooms with healing gardens. This is the work of Annette Ridenour, an arts and healthcare pioneer who has worked for more than thirty-five years developing arts programs for healthcare institutions around the United States. Her work in the design of harmonic environments and sacred space heals people deeply and spiritually while they are in her healing hospital environments, and her work training artists in a variety of healthcare settings expands the practice of healing art at the bedside.

Annette believes that the intention embedded in the art experience, whether it is visual, performing, or participative, is transformative to the viewer/participant. That is why she creates her hospital environments with love, joy, and the intention of healing or opening. Her intentionally healing spiritual environments are a catalyst for personal growth and transcendence, not only for the artist but also for those who experience the art. Art meets people wherever they are and takes them on a personal journey that is theirs alone. The arts are also a great storyteller. We know our past through viewing the art of past civilizations. Annette encourages us to tell our stories through art—our individual stories and stories from our family, our community, and our culture. The healing stories and personal myths resonate with our spiritual DNA and connect people to generations past to heal deeply. Annette is a powerful force in changing hospitals to become intentional healing spiritual environments.

Annette Ridenour, a world leader in hospital design and art and medicine program implementation, talks about designing and creating hospital environments that intentionally promote a space that heals and cares. http://www.youtube.com/watch?v=UyrWBkmwFrI&list=PLMm-0ccB -CYpmKktLEws7WlrNyNg2QDnu&index=4

## *Exercises for Protection*

Many healers have the experience of feeling symptoms like those of the person they are treating. Some even use this for diagnosis when they understand and can control this phenomenon. The healer will feel the symptom in their body and know what needs healing; then they knew how to let it go and to not be afraid but continue to feel it. When you are doing healing work and you focus on the negative, doing the healing from your personality, you can absorb the illness in your body, but there's a secret to keeping yourself from burning out: If you release yourself to a higher consciousness—whether it is God, a bear spirit, an angel, or your inner creativity—you tap into the infinite source of energy that all healing comes from.

Healers have traditionally used spiritual tools like this to protect themselves from negative energy when they do healings. These are old secrets passed down through the ages by spiritual healers to protect themselves by harnessing the energy of a higher consciousness to flow through them. The energy or spirit of the illness can often be neutralized by higher healing energy. This avoids compassion fatigue or burnout and protects the healer from taking on the illness of the person they are working with. The traditional Native American view of this was that the spirits that caused illness would leave the person being healed and go to the Creator, not the healer. In this way, the healer protects themselves by healing with the power of higher consciousness, not with their own body.

In this view, a surgeon is an instrument of a higher force. Their will is their own, but the passion to heal ultimately comes from beyond a higher consciousness. The intention to heal facilitates greater energy to come through them. Similarly, when you tap into a higher source correctly, it can energize you, not deplete you—you don't absorb a person's negative story and get horribly sick afterward. Instead, you allow the flow of a universal spirit to take it away. When healing artists are connected to a higher level of being, it's not about themselves personally. The art brings the higher consciousness to light. The higher consciousness does the healing.

You are a spirit-filled person. To heal, align yourself with the eternal wellspring that flows through you. It is spirit being revealed. You tap into a source with greater power than yourself.

Healers have many ways of protection. All the ways rely on a higher consciousness to take the illness or create a field of protection. They can use guided imagery, pray to a Higher Power, make a bubble or shield, build a fire so the illness can go to the Creator, light sage, use herbs or cornmeal to take the energy, or make a story where the illness goes to a spirit animal or helper who does the healing. We have exercises in the praxis section for protection if you feel this is an important part of healing.

Let the healing energy of the nonjudgmental higher consciousness of love flow through you. Heal with that energy. Whatever you decide your imaginary vehicle for higher consciousness is, whatever culture or religion you wish to draw from, let your spirit, spirit guides, and spirit animals do the healing. Get out of the way and don't let your personality do the healing. In your mind's eye, let the higher consciousness create a protective shield around you.

Make a prayer for protection. Pray that what needs to stay out of the circle for healing will stay out and that what needs to be in the ring will come in. Pray that the higher consciousness of love comes into you and does the healing, takes the illness, and neutralizes it.

## Working with the Environment and the Earth

We are part of the physical realm, a thread in the tapestry of life on this planet. We are part of the cycles of the earth itself, and we can help re-establish balance on the planet. It reflects healing with each one of us. We are part of the creative environment of the earth. Our bodies are as beautiful as the most beautiful flower. We have innate intelligence of deep healing forms. We are of the earth, and the earth is creative. Creativity is sacred, generated by an infinite field of love and the life force within ourselves.

- Change your environment: your house, garden, bedroom, a new place.
- Create a community garden.
- Clean up garbage as an art piece; clean the water, land, mountain, beach, and sea.
- Make a huge environmental installation; plant trees or put lightning rods in a circle.

### Artist-Healer Profile: Betsy Damon—Keeper of the Water

Forty years ago, Betsy Damon stepped outside her traditional art training and carved a unique path to work with the environment, communities, science, and art. She began looking to her inner consciousness as a source of inspiration, which initiated her public engagement, starting with gritty art performances on New York City streets. She was engaged in the women's movement of the 1970s when she founded No Limits for Women in the Arts, a network to join and support female artists.

In 1985, after a cross-country camping trip with her children, Betsy found herself reconnected to the primal elements of the natural world—the sound of wind, the flow of water, the forest, the rain. This initiated the casting of a 250-foot dry riverbed, *The Memory of Clean Water*, which brought her attention to the invisible destruction that development was having on water sources. In the early evening, while casting the riverbed, Betsy looked up to realize that the stones of the riverbed were patterned like the stars of the sky. The patterns of water were everywhere. She committed herself to learning everything about water. Little did she know that twenty-seven years later she would still be deeply entrenched.

Beginning with the creation of Keepers of the Waters in 1991, Betsy has continued to work toward creating community-based models of water stewardship. Her work includes sculpture, teaching, lectures and workshops. In China she created the nation's first public art event for the environment and, most notably, the Living Water Garden, a world-renowned public park and natural water filtration model. In the United States, she continuously works with communities and grassroots groups and completes art/design commissions.

Betsy's inspiration comes from extensive research of sacred water sites, and her curiosity for the biology and earth sciences that compose living systems. Always seeking new ways to articulate the complexity of water and engage communities in caring for this precious resource, Betsy continues her passion.

 *Water Rules Life*, a visual art media piece by environmental artist and activist Betsy Damon, shows how art heals environments.
http://www.youtube.com/watch?v=7HdYhzjMnQk&list=PLMm-OccB
-CYpmKktLEws7WlrNyNg2QDnu&index=3

## *Media to Consider for Your Final Medicine Art Project*

- What art making did you love as a child?
- Visual arts: photography, painting, watercolors, drawings, sculpture, Play-Doh, film, huge sculptures, assemblages, puppets, masks, painted skateboards, jewelry, ceramics
- Words: poetry, short stories, novels, theater, puppets, plays, imaginary playmates, characters, monologues, webinars, films with interviews
- Music: singing, listening, making an album of songs you love, chanting, playing an instrument, toning, bowls, drumming, going to nature for sounds
- Dancing: doing a dance for peace, dancing with patients, participating in large dances for social change
- Ceremony: going to church; evoking visions, spirits, spirit animals; making medicine wheels, huge medicine wheel; pilgrimages; building a chapel

## *More Examples of Final Medicine Art Projects and Presentations*

- A man worked with students in a special school for troubled youth. He had the children make photos of their essence, showed us the photographs, and told the stories about the children.
- A woman made a sacred hut for healing in a home for children with severe behavioral and social problems. She showed us photographs of the hut and told the stories of children coming into it.
- A mother and daughter made a book together with collages and reflections. The daughter brought the book to class and shared it.
- A woman made a quilt to heal a friend with breast cancer. She brought the quilt to class.
- For her boyfriend who had committed suicide, a woman made a healing garden made from junkyard items. She cleaned, planted, and dug out the backyard to make a memorial garden. She shared photographs and a film of her work.
- A woman made a bench to meditate in her backyard. It required a full cleaning, planting, and renewal process. She shared photographs.
- A man made ceramic bowls as gifts for patients' families in the hospital. He brought some bowls to show and took pictures of the families.
- A woman crafted handmade stuffed animals for children in a children's hospital. She brought some of her work to class.
- A woman made a life-sized self-portrait with oil paints. She brought her paintings and shared them.
- Many people have made a memory book for grandparents who died. They bring their book, pass it around, and tell the story of their family and love.
- A woman did interviews about happiness with all her female relatives over the age of fifty years. She talked to all her aunts and grandmothers. She read the interviews to us.
- A woman listen to a woman dying in a hospice tell her life story and wrote the story of her life for her family.
- A man made video interviews with breast cancer patients discussing what they thought about dying.
- A woman went on a three-day vision quest and wrote about it in her journal.

- A woman made a huge medicine wheel with her boyfriend for a baby they'd lost in a miscarriage. He took photographs and gave them to her to show his love for her.
- A woman made photographs of her own body to not to be critical of herself. She made beautiful photographs to see her own beauty.
- A woman asked her boyfriend to paint her body with henna, to heal her memory of scoliosis surgery. He painted her back straight and beautiful.
- A woman asked all her friends to paint henna mandalas all over her body to make her beautiful. She was so beautiful to everyone.

## Final Medicine Art Projects about Sexuality and Body Image

- A pregnant woman painting the earth on her belly and becoming an earth mother
- A woman performing a piece from *The Vagina Monologues* about orgasms
- A woman painting a life-sized illustration of her naked body and letting it tell its new story
- A woman making a painting of her body in a life-size tracing, and telling the story of all its energies
- A woman casting her torso in plaster to heal feelings about her breasts
- A man creating a book of paintings about sexual abuse
- A dance to heal rape
- Participants creating self-portraits of looking beautiful to heal sexual abuse memories see themselves as gods or goddesses. They enhance femininity and sexual self.

## Final Medicine Art Projects About Death

Since we began sharing the art-healing process, there have been many, many final Medicine Art projects about death. Here are some examples:

- Making a memorial garden. A young college student did her final Medicine Art project to grieve the suicide of her ex-boyfriend. She had done a lot of grieving but wanted to move forward in her life. She wanted to create a new perspective on his death. She had just moved into a new house. The backyard was a junk-filled trash pile. She decided to make a garden there as a memorial for him. She had never made a garden before and did not know anything about the process. It took all her physical labor. She cleared and packed years of trash. She got her hands dirty. It took her two weeks just to take out the garbage. Then she got soil; bought books about gardens; asked questions; and learned more about nutrients, plants, and fertilizers. The work was so physical and arduous, it became an incredible experience dedicated to the memory of her ex-boyfriend. Out of her garden came new life, positivity, and growth. It was a deeply healing experience for her to work through her grief to move past this painful time.

- A project to grieve the death of a mother, done by her daughter and grandchildren. The daughter made a sacred circle next to the sea, in her mother's favorite place. She led her family in a walk around it and then she showed slides of her mother in her home. She did this a year after her mother's death as her final Medicine Art project. Nothing had been done to memorialize her mother's death. She filmed the ceremony for her project. While she showed the film to the class, she served her mother's favorite food.

- A daughter did a memorial PowerPoint for her mother and told the story of her mother's life. She showed beautiful photographs of her mother and her family then she led prayers for her mother's passing over.

- A woman spent a whole day on a mountain in winter, making a sacred circle with stone to grieve the loss of an unborn baby. All day, she moved large rocks herself and made a circle that looked like a medicine wheel of Native American people. She had not done anything before to memorialize her loss. She shared this powerful work with the class with slides taken by her lover. As we watched them we could see how much he loved her as she made art to grieve in sacred space.

- A woman had painful images of her brother's death that she could not get rid of. She did guided imagery and art to see the death and her brother in a new way. She played his favorite music, showed slides of him and his friends, and re-storyed her memory of his death. This was very powerful: she had been haunted by images of a violent death, but with guided imagery and art, she replaced them with images of his beauty, friends, work, and life.

## How to Share Your Final Medicine Art Project

Part of your healing with art is sharing your art with another person, in an intentional community of love, nonjudgment, support, and even prayer. When we do the Art as a Healing Force process with groups, we do this from the first day. It strengthens the process greatly.

We invite your sharing to take place in a field of protection. This is a new experience for most people. We are used to being judgmental when we listen to others. In a university, most classes are about grading, performance, and technical skill. Our art-healing classes and workshops are a fundamentally different experience. People are not graded on skill in their art at all. We tell people we work with that art for healing is about process, meaning, and transformation. Leave your Inner Critic at the door when you come in to present; listen, especially to yourself. Listen with love, see beauty, listen with compassion and caring, and accept what you hear as perfect. The sharing is a gift of love and healing to your self, others, community, and the earth. Imagine how beautiful it is to be your authentic self in a field of infinite love. This is what it is like to present your final medicine art project to someone.

## Preparing for Your Presentation

Make a fifteen-minute presentation of your final Medicine Art project. In your presentation, share what you wanted to heal, the art process you used, and what happened. Then share your actual project. Dance, show your paintings and talk about them, play music, read poetry, read your journal, show a PowerPoint about what you did, show photographs of what you did, and share your art and healing experience with someone.

Even if you share only with yourself, the presentation is an important part of the twelve-week art-healing experience. Presenting the project makes it real. You are a witness to your healing by speaking about it and showing it; your work takes on another level of power. If you share with another person, it is more profound. The person witnesses your project with love and care; you are seen truly as who you are.

The presentation is actually a ceremony. It's not a performance; it's a prayer. It is a gift to you and to the people you present to. For many people who do our process, the presentation and the witnessing of the presentations is the most powerful part of the whole twelve weeks. Often, the day or days are full of love, tears, caring, and compassion. It is unbelievable and more beautiful than anyone expects.

## Part Three: Sacred Ceremony with Art to Heal

Ceremony puts it all together. It closes the circle of art and healing. Ceremony is visual arts, word, dance, and music done all together, at one time, with the intent to make sacred space and to heal. It is that simple. That is why our twelve-week program includes so much ceremony—it is a way to concentrate the energy and focus intent on creating the space for healing. It's an intentional, ritualistic process using all the art media together to heal yourself, others, your community, or the earth. It is the oldest form of healing and the oldest form of art. A ceremony is as powerful as any medicine we have to heal body, mind, and spirit.

Since ancient times, ceremony is a most powerful way to illuminate spirit. It ties together the golden threads of this book by helping you make your own ceremony to illuminate your spirit more brightly.

### Layla's Story: It's Not a Performance; It's a Prayer

Layla, a Chumash Indian woman from Southern California, was about to do the butterfly dance for a large group of people as part of a healing ceremony. She was an elder, with wrinkles honoring her age. She was dressed as a beautiful butterfly. Her children and grandchildren surrounded her, all dressed as butterflies; the youngest was only about five years old. They stood patiently in a line in the dance circle in front of the people who were outside the ring.

Layla stood and spoke. "I will do the butterfly dance now for you, with my family. We are honored to be here. I want to tell you something first: It's not a performance; it's a prayer."

When her grandson, the drummer, hit the drum with his drumsticks, the circle came alive. The small children went in and out from the edges of their line to the center of the circle as butterfly spirits. It was so beautiful to watch. They fluttered around with their small wings, seemingly floating off the ground. They danced and brought in the butterfly spirit, healing the whole group. As they danced, you could feel the faint flapping of the butterfly wings on your body, taking away what needed to leave and putting in pure innocent grace.

It's interesting that our culture calls this mixture of visual art, music, dance, and word "performance art." But for us, as artist-healers, it is a not a performance; it's a prayer, like Layla said. In healing with the arts, a ceremony has the intention to heal, not just for performance's sake. The difference is why you are doing what you do and what you are praying for. What is in your heart when you dance? The difference between prayer and performance art is crucial to understand what we do as artist-healers. Remember the story of the woman who wanted to protect her daughter from soldiers? That was not a performance to entertain the class. It was a ceremony to heal this woman and her family; a ceremony to heal a story that had poisoned her life, her culture, and her soul. This is different. This is prayer.

## Intimate Personal Ceremonies

A small, intimate, personal ritual is a good way to bring ceremony into your life. A ceremony can be as simple as a daily prayer and meditation practice in a sacred space. To do this, you simply create a healing environment you can drop into. Your simple practice may be lighting a candle and then practicing deep breathing. Mary does a ceremony when she wakes up for her intimate morning ritual. She described it like this:

I ring my singing bowls three times and then my Tibetan bells. I turn my prayer wheel slowly, praying for my intentions of the day. My altar has a Buddha, a statue of the Virgin Mary, and sacred objects from around the world. I make a prayer to create intention to be with the Creator's presence in my life. I do this with God, the greater spirit, Jesus, the Virgin Mary, and Buddha, all combined into a sacred higher consciousness. Each day, I ask for guidance and wisdom to manifest in each moment of my life and to allow the mystery of the day to unfold. I pray to honor others and for forgiveness for myself and others. This small ceremony in the beginning of my day grounds me in my life, creating a pattern of being that brings peace and comfort. I use ceremony to be creative.

When I engage in it, I am making art. It uses all senses. When I work with a group of people, it is ceremony. Each meeting of my class is a ceremonial gathering that creates protection and a time and space where deep work can be done.

## *Larger Group Ceremonies*

You can also do larger ceremonies with groups of people for healing. These ceremonies are very powerful and fun. In the last class of her twelve-week process, Mary does a group fire ceremony that is a favorite with people who have taken the class. It is very simple. She makes a fire and invites people to stand up and tell the story of what they want to let go of and then throw it into the fire. For example, one person says, "I am putting this huge rope in the fire. It bound me, made my burden. I want to release myself from all my obligations. I want to release myself from taking care of my family and other people. I want to take care of myself now." People bring all kinds of stuff: old books, love letters, journals, furniture, and other mementos. One person said, "This is all my data from my PhD. It's finished now, and I want to let it go." Another person might say, "I will tell a story I have never told—as I tell it, I throw it into the fire." Everyone watches the items being burned. Fire engulfs them, burning these offerings. They are gone; they disappear. At the end, the group has a celebration to bring in lightness with singing, drumming, and guitar music for the whole community.

In terms of your twelve-week process for this book, you can do a fire ceremony in many ways. You can do a guided imagery, in your mind's eye throwing something into a fire. You can do the ceremony alone with a small fire, your fireplace, or even a candle, actually burning what you want to let go of. You can make a big fire with others who are doing the art and healing process and make your own ceremony to let go of something in your life. Finally, you can make a big ceremony that is open and invite people, to make it healing for your community.

### Examples of Group Ceremonies

A ceremony to

- Make an art and healing piece with dancers, musicians, and poets
- Bring in the light with a group of people
- Graduate from the art and healing process
- Honor someone who has died

- Let go of things you don't want anymore
- Heal with dance
- Heal a river, mountain, or other area from violence

## Margi's Story: Throwing Away Things from a Toxic Relationship

Margi did the Art as a Healing Force process as part of her graduate work in arts and transformation. She was an experienced artist and had spent many semesters doing art for consciousness transformation. Her project was a personal ceremony to help her daughter get rid of a boyfriend and move on in her life. To heal, you need to get rid of what needs to go, make a change in your life, and then actually change.

Margi told us about it.

I chose this project for art and healing and found myself wildly enthusiastic about the process. I have experienced the healing power of art in many forms within my own life and was interested in taking what I have learned and seeing how it would work with others.

The project was with my daughter. She has spent several years healing from an extremely toxic relationship. She felt that she was nearing the end of that process and wanted to make her healing tangible. She wanted to do something incorporating the idea of the natural elements.

First, she made a box containing some personal effects from the man with whom she had had a long relationship. She covered the box with poetry he had written to her and some of her own drawings. As she thought about this, she became convinced that she wanted to burn it.

She asked my husband and me to participate with her in a ritual of burning the box and saying a few words to acknowledge the importance of this person in her life and the destruction he'd brought, as well as breaking the power he had in her life. She had written a few pages of renunciation, which she read as the box burned. This brought her a tremendous sense of release, freedom, and joy. She felt at this moment that her process of healing was finished.

She carefully took the ashes home with her and waited until we talked further. The next step became clear. For her second event in the healing process, she wanted to do a Chinese brush painting of the characters for *death* and *joy*.

She mixed some of the ashes into the ink; the result was a gritty texture, not un-reminiscent of bones from cremation. This pleased her greatly, as it gave a sense of finality to the aspects of the relationship she was healing from.

The final step took place several weeks later. I had been making cairns at Pt. Isabel. She asked to join me and construct a funeral cairn to bury the ashes in. She used a lovely triangulated group of rusty wire as a base. She built her cairn out of composite riprap. It was important to her to use discarded building materials in the place of natural stones to further symbolize the ending of the control this person had held over her and the destruction he had brought into her life. She poured the ashes into the cairn and finished the construction with stones on the top as adornments.

The following day when we went back, there had been two high tides since the cairn had been built. The tide was still up, though not high. The cairn was partially submerged and the ashes were covered with water. She was struck by the image of the tide rising and very gently carrying the ashes of this relationship out to sea. I was honored to have been her companion through this process. I felt that as she did, she had come to a place of rest. She felt released from the pain that had defined her for several years. She was ready to move forward into new, healthy relationships.

This process was a natural one for me as we had talked extensively over the course of this process about what she might do to celebrate the end of this step in her process of healing. She was easy to work with, in great part because of our closeness and the love and trust we have for each other.

## Lessons from Margi's Project

- The art-healing process evolves naturally.
- Healing happens in natural, heartfelt steps.
- You can facilitate healing with someone you love using art and ceremony.
- Healing is about love and relationship.
- Art and healing is natural.
- Art and healing is a sacred ceremony.
- The process is fun, deep, hard, intense, heartfelt, and wonderful.
- Healing beings family together in love and trust.

## Troy's Story: Finding a Whole New Perspective on Life

I believe that my project awakened parts of me that had been sleeping for some time. It gave me a whole new perspective on life. I learned what it was like to live more intuitively in the flow of life, rather than within a strict schedule. Currently, I am taking classes to become a minister with Centers for Spiritual Living; it's something I really love. I also practice yoga, meditate, dance, play, explore, and create with different art forms regularly. It has become a way of life for me. Living this way, I have found a community of people with similar views and priorities—to live creatively, authentically, and with care for themselves and the world as a whole.

I feel connected with myself and have these amazing tools that help me settle into myself and see clearly where I want to go and what I want to do. These tools are art, movement, prayer, and meditation. I find that just by setting an intention, creating space and time to be in the moment with one of these activities, and then allowing the process to unfold, I receive what I had intended.

Constantly returning to myself is my practice, whether I find myself in a grounding breath, sitting still, after lots of movement and dance, in painting, or just letting go and crying. It's like a layer is shed each time and I see again, and feel again, my self. My journey is seeing who I am. I feel closer to myself all the time—more real, more authentic—and I am surrounded by people who are also returning to themselves.

It's much easier than it seems. Anyone can do it. I've felt my own transformations happen in minutes and also over months. I've seen people renewed after one evening of creating art. It's simple, and it's so fun! Art in Healing is one of my passions, along with yoga—both create sacred space for people to come alive in beautiful and deep ways.

# Week 12 Praxis

This final guided imagery of the book is your graduation ceremony. We do it as an initiation so you can fully own your new self as an artist-healer. We honor your new self. We end this book by creating a sacred personal space to honor you with a ceremony of proclamation. In this ceremony, we want to honor you as new artist-healer, anoint you, and initiate you into the beautiful creative process that you participated in.

## Guided Imagery: Your Initiation as an Artist-Healer

To begin, imagine yourself in a place that feels comfortable and safe. Focus on your heart and move into a still point within yourself. Imagine your tension dissolving, allowing yourself to move into a place within which you feel centered, open, and relaxed. In your mind's eye, breathe into the area around your heart. As you relax, feel your body letting go.

Now we are going to take you on a journey. Imagine you're walking down a beautiful path in the country. As you walk, you feel the breeze on your body and the sunlight on your skin. You smell the forest. You are so quiet in this moment that you can almost hear the grass growing. We invite you to feel a deep sense of peacefulness. Know that you have always been on the right path. You are exactly where you need to be in life right now. Your life has brought you to this moment in time. The experience and memories of your life are uniquely yours. Your life is a creative and transformative experience. You are walking into the center of yourself.

Now, imagine you are walking toward a sacred circle. You can imagine a circle of stones, a circle of ancient trees, or even a circle of stars. In your mind's eye, invite people who love you and work with you to come into the circle. This is a ceremony of graduation, a ceremony of initiation to your new life as an artist-healer. Invite friends, family, loved ones, and ancestors to this moment of your initiation. Now imagine you are walking in a ceremonial procession to enter the circle. As you enter the circle, you see that this group is ready to receive and honor you. As you see this in your mind's eye, know that it's real. This is actually happening.

Stand in the center of the circle with your loved ones and teachers around you. As you stand in the circle, see that it is a safe and sacred place. Look around. What do you see? Who is here with you now? Go to the center of the circle. Feel your connection to the earth and the infinite space and sky above you. Know that this work is a gentle, loving, compassionate energy. You are embraced with total acceptance, kindness, and gentleness. Listen with your heart.

Now imagine in your mind's eye that we're walking up to you. We are standing in front of you, welcoming you with open arms. We offer you this gift: the realization of you as an artist-healer. Imagine your body filling up with an extraordinary, beautiful light. As the light comes into you, you are fulfilled as an artist. Feel yourself being this artist. You are creative, strong, and illuminated. Imagine this part of you opening a vortex of energy that empowers you to be the artist you truly are. Experience the radiance and creative energy pulsating through your whole body. You are already an artist and always have been. This is a reminder, a confirmation, initiating you into being who you truly are. You have walked this journey of creativity. This is your gift; it has always been within you. In your mind's eye, honor the memories of the art you have made in these twelve weeks. Remember what you have done and how it has changed your life.

Now we have something else to tell you. We tell you that you are a healer. Your body can heal itself from illness. Your immune system is strong; you can make new cells when you are injured. You can heal from wounds, surgery, and infections. You have an Inner Healer who has evolved over a million years within you who is strong and powerful. This healer evolved to keep you well and to heal you from illness.

Now we tell you to look inside yourself. The Inner Artist and the Inner Healer have become one. You have accomplished the transformative merging of these two powerful energies within you. As you see who you have become, proclaim these words in the silence of your mind. Speak them out loud. It is your proclamation of yourself as an artist-healer: "I am an artist. I am a healer. I am an artist-healer." Again: "I am an artist. I am a healer. I am an artist-healer." Again: "I am an artist. I am a healer. I am an artist-healer." The spirit of this book gives this to you as a mantra. Take it into your heart.

Now say the second mantra: "I am an artist. I am a healer. The artist and healer are one." Again, say, "I am an artist. I am a healer. The artist and healer are one." And again, "I am an artist. I am a healer. The artist and healer are one." Fully experience the emergence of these energies within you. Feel the artist and healer who have awakened in each of your cells. See them as one powerful, radiant body you are carrying.

Receive this gift and your proclamation in your essence. The gift is a message of who you truly are. Now allow us to dissolve into the landscape. Say good-bye and know that we will always to be with you and support you, wherever you are. Take a few minutes to be in the center of this circle. Experience yourself fully as the embodied artist and the healer. This moment is deeply real and personal.

When you are ready, return to the forest path. This time you are radiant, shining with light from within. You are now an awakened artist-healer. When you make art, you are tapping into the great healing force that resides within you. Now relax and fully integrate this experience in your body.

 Mary leads an Art as a Healing Force graduation ceremony and blessing. http://www.youtube.com/watch?v=ehYGTFD8pE4&feature=youtu.be

To complete your twelve-week process, you can do this exercise as a guided imagery. You can tell someone in your life that you are an artist-healer; or you can make a circle with friends doing the process and make your declaration: "I am an artist. I am a healer. I am an artist-healer," to the whole group. You can also do this on the internet or in your art-healing group. When you speak the words, they have power; you own the role. You are the artist-healer. As you say the words, you acknowledge your power to yourself and a group. It is a declaration, a proclamation, an owning, and a statement of who you are now in your changed life. It is very powerful to say these words in front of a group. Everyone sees you as an artist-healer, and you see yourself as an artist-healer.

## Summary of Week 12

- Do the guided imagery to experience transcendence.
- Do the Medicine Art to bring in the light.
- Work with another person as an artist-healer.
- Complete and share your final Medicine Art project with yourself or others.
- Do the guided imagery for the final ceremony, "I am an artist-healer."

# CONCLUSION: CREATIVE LUMINOSITY

*In the beginning it was a secret; now, it is a gift.*
*The gift of who we are is ours to give, and only we can give it.*
*May we be blessed in life and bless others in work*
*as we bring love and healing into expression.*

This book has been an invitation for you to learn about how to use Art as a Healing Force and become part of the artist-healer community just by practicing art and healing.

In your life, we hope you return to this work we've started together. We hope you use art to heal over and over again. As you experience art and healing, you will realize that it is not a linear process but, rather, a spiral. We usually start in the beginning with darkness, move to transcendence, spiral back to darkness, and start again. As you heal, going around and around, you may return to certain parts of the cycle many times in your lifetime. Each time, your experience will deepen. May this book be a guiding light for you on your path of healing and continue to help and accompany you on this journey as you use creativity to find out what needs to be healed and embody who you truly are.

Healing with art is a natural process. In many ways it is as simple as breathing. It frees an internal life force that is automatic, like your heartbeat. This is the eternal wellspring of creativity, living, breathing, being alive in every minute of your life, and pumping creativity thorough your body. This is the healing force, the life rhythm we're all tied to.

Just as everyone is a healer, everyone has an Inner Artist. We create ourselves, the world we live in, our homes, our food, our gardens, our family, our circles of friends, and our bodies. Create love with your thoughts, words, and actions.

At the same time, your body is filled with incredible wisdom and light. You are part of an infinite field of creativity. Each person is like a star in the night sky. There are billions of us, all sharing art and healing, getting together to make art to heal ourselves, others, our community, or the earth. Each is beautiful, a human star, a shining artist-healer. You are one point of unique, luminous consciousness. Let your light shine by being who you are.

Know, too, that you are not alone in this world. Perhaps you've been able to connect more with your fellow artist-healers in your group. Or you're now ready to find out more about one of the featured artist-healers in the book. Whatever the case may be, when you leave this circle, know that there are many people in your community who can support you in this way.

Having graduated from the art-healing program, you are an artist-healer. You can make art to heal your life, another person's life, the community you live in, or the earth. You can change the world you live in, or you can heal illnesses, emotional problems, and initiate spiritual growth for yourself and people around you. You can start a group and bring this program to your church, hospital, elder care center, school, and more. You can become a facilitator of art and healing and lead classes to teach others this work. As we have shown, there are no limits to what you can do.

*You are the artist-healer we've been waiting for.*

# ACKNOWLEDGMENTS

## From Michael

I thank sculptor James Surls for my vision of art and healing as one, Linda Samuels for cofounding Art as a Healing Force, Marion Weber for supporting our work at Art as a Healing Force, Michael Lerner at Commonweal for supporting the Art as a Healing Force annual conferences, Annette Ridenhour and Society of Arts in Healthcare for a family of art and healing, Kenn Burrows and Adam Burke at the San Francisco State University Institute for Holistic Health Studies for supporting my course, and Karen Sjoholm at John F. Kennedy University Transformative Arts program. I thank my patients and the people I have worked with for their wonderful visions and stories. And finally, my family: Rudy; Lewis; and my granddaughters, Lucy, Roya, Mauren, and Nicola. You are the center of my life.

# From Mary

Thank you to the Shands Arts in Medicine program and all the wonderful individuals who bring this work to patients, staff, and families, as well as the College of Nursing and the Center of Spirituality and Health, for supporting my academic work. I want to acknowledge my colleagues in the Watson Caring Science Institute, especially Tarron Estes and Marilyn Fogerty. I want to acknowledge Emi Lenes for her constant love and support and Cathy Dewitt for her contribution to this field. I appreciate Beyond Words for the cocreation of this book. I want to thank Harold Nobles for his videos, Thom Golia for his incredible photography, and Inna Dagman for her dancing Goddess. I want to thank all my students who have taken my class over the years, and all the friends I do not even know who have contributed to this work by bringing the arts into healing. I honor the beautiful work of everyone all over the world who share this vision. Most of all, I thank my family: Tim, Anneliese, David, and Francesco.

Together, we would both like to thank all our students who have taken our courses for their brilliant projects and inspiration; and all the artists in art and healing for a life of wonder. We would also like thank each other as coauthors for cocreating and co-channeling this work, and the people at Beyond Words.